Profound Meaning

Oncology Clinicians Share Their Insight

Sarah F. Kurker
Arizona State University

innovativeink
PUBLISHING
A Division of Kendall Hunt

innovativeink PUBLISHING
A Division of Kendall Hunt

www.kendallhunt.com
Send all inquiries to:
4050 Westmark Drive
Dubuque, IA 52004-1840

ISBN: 979-8-3851-5994-9

Published in the United States of America

Dedication

I have had the incredible experience of working with some dedicated, caring, and intelligent colleagues over my years in oncology social work. These individuals have inspired me to be the best I can be for my patients.

Choosing oncology social work was my passion and meaning in my life, and I cherish my interactions with my patients and their families. My patients have impacted me in a way that words can't always capture. But the moments, good and really hard, have made me who I am. It has inspired me to be influential not only in my field and in the field of social work but also in my teaching. I incorporate those experiences, feelings, and lessons in the teaching I do at Arizona State University (ASU) in Social Work and Integrative Health.

On a personal level, while it is sad and unexplainable why children have to go through cancer, I am thankful that I can be present with people during such really hard times. I value that they allow me to be there with them in such meaningful times.

I would like to thank Emily and Evan for my greatest love as your mom. I am always here for you. Kevin, I appreciate you. Mom and Dad thank you for giving me my education which has been a great foundation of the work I do. Thanks, to my sister Cindy, for always supporting me.

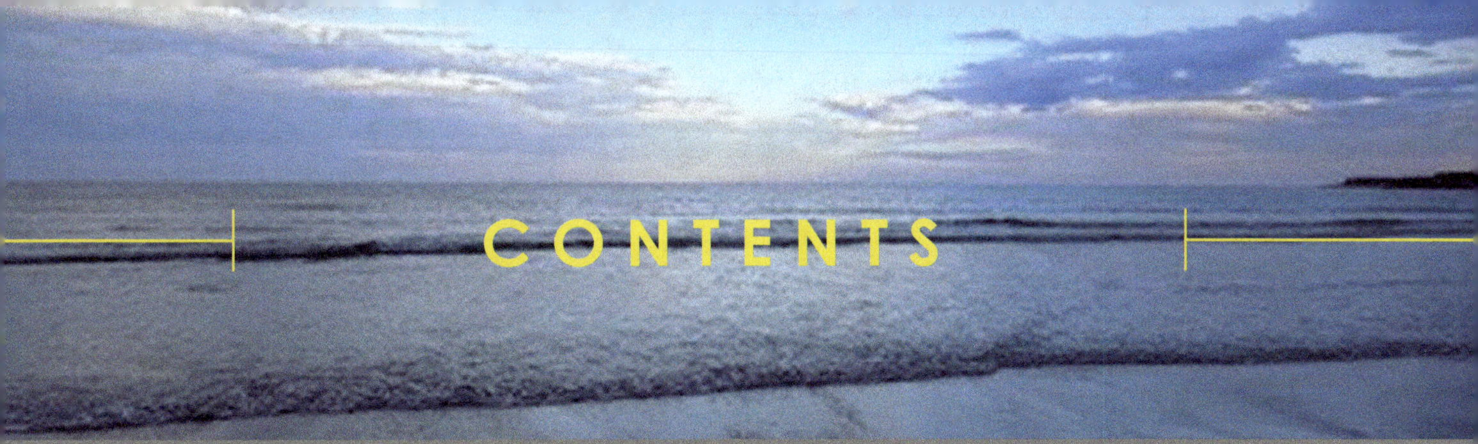

CONTENTS

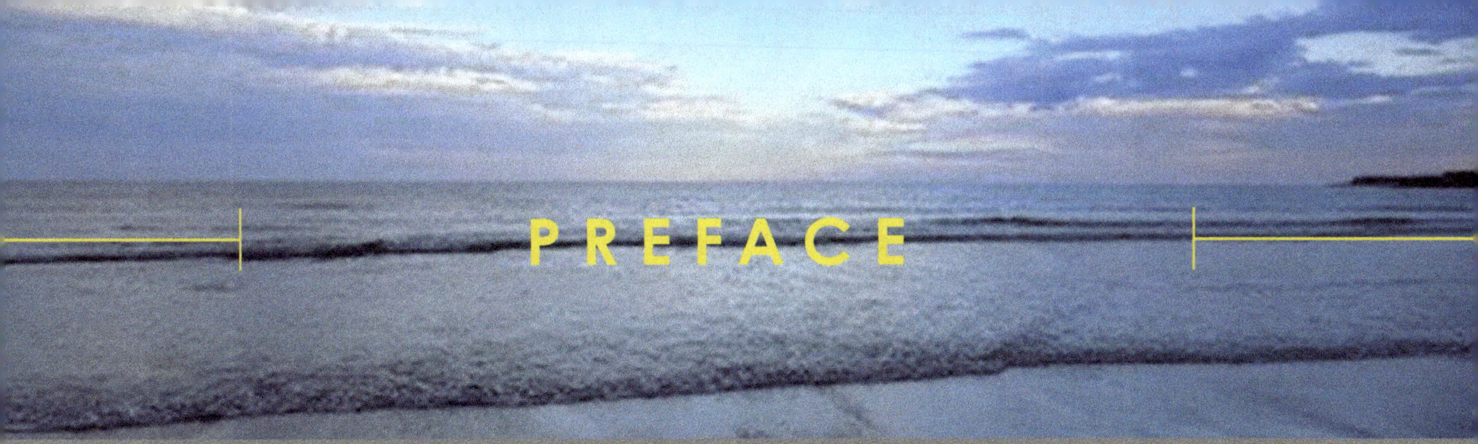

PREFACE

As an oncology social worker for my entire career I have been fortunate to support patients during a really challenging time in their lives. Because enduring cancer is so intense, my connection to patients and their families is profound. These moments have impacted me in all that I do. I know this work is so meaningful. I feel fortunate to have chosen this career and learn from my patients. My patients' experiences and stories strengthen my ability to provide integrative care. It has enabled me to be a faculty instructor to share the wisdom of these experiences. I have been fortunate to start my career at Boston Children's Hospital. I have worked at the Arizona Cancer Center and Banner University in Tucson, Arizona. I then had the incredible experience of being an integral part of Massachusetts General Hospital Cancer Center.

As a social work intern at the Arizona Cancer Center, I was an American Cancer Society Trainer and I was able to create my first cancer support group. I noticed a theme in my patients; young parents diagnosed with cancer needed additional support, not so much on the cancer, but how to parent with cancer. I have facilitated many groups since observing and learning. The group dynamic in social work is pretty incredible. The reciprocity that flows in a group is impactful as they support each other. And to be able to facilitate that support it is magical in grief and in hope. Every job I have had, I have incorporated groups based on the needs of my patients. I have been fortunate to do a young adult support group. I have also been able to lead meditation and visualization groups. I created a group for parents of children with cancer. Developing and facilitating these groups has been influential in my understanding of supporting patients.

My most impactful role was being the pediatric bone marrow transplant social worker. This was my first job with my master's degree. The children and families really went through hell and just tried to survive. To witness this trauma and be consistently supportive for them made me a stronger person. There are so many families that have left me with ongoing memories, hard and inspiring. I will always value being able to do this work.

I also had the privilege to be a senior research specialist at the Arizona Cancer Center, focusing on quality-of-life research for oncology patients. Then came the unexpected opportunity to learn about program development and the impact of psychosocial supports for my patients. I was able to connect the impact of publishing. When you are able to publish your work, others can develop similar programs and inspiration. That connection to impact oncology care is significant. This experience impacted my career by always providing evidence-based practice. It also reassured me that visions and changes I wanted to make for my patients were accessible.

I am honored to have elevated my career in teaching at Arizona State University (ASU), where I proudly graduated with my master's degree in social work. To be able to incorporate my clinical oncology skills to inspire students to learn curriculum really connects my passion of evidence-based interventions. I find meaning to be able to inspire social work students to make positive changes in their communities. In my role as a faculty instructor, I am inspired by my students and the work they do in the social work field.

When I reflect back on these moments of finding professional and personal meaning in my work, I know the foundation is mindfulness. My discovery of dedicating my career and impact in oncology was created in a mindful realization. And not only has it directed me to the passion of my work, I have also been able to learn, practice, and teach mindfulness to my patients and students. Developing meaning in this work connects me in a mindful way.

I try to encourage others to make their job personal. Adding things that bring you joy and exposing your clients to them allow for growth and development for all impacted.

Another aspect of my individual career is to bring in my passions. For me, movement is the foundation of my being. I love to be active and incorporate being present in my social work career too. When I was the pediatric bone marrow social worker, I saw how parents were just inactive watching their kids go through this pain. I found that instead of meeting with them in the hospital, we would do our therapy out walking (when we had someone they trusted to be with their child). We would walk around the hospital, and just getting outdoors and moving was therapeutic for them. I teach this to my clients and my students because there are so many important benefits to moving. I would try to get siblings passes to the gym so they had some time alone in movement. I know the benefit of moving and wanted my patients and families to have that outlet.

I love to buy things that would bring happiness to my patients. I would never let them know it was from me but was donated. It would give them a smile or a distraction from what they had. I spent time getting donations so that families could have some family time outside of cancer. I wanted them to have a meal out or go get ice cream. Many of the families had financial limitations, so I wrote a grant to get funding to give them these special memories.

I love capturing moments of beauty through photography. I incorporate this into my interventions by taking photos of nature and then sending a note or quote to my patients who are going through a hard time. It may bring them some joy and support outside of our interventions. Creating supports for others in my art is meaningful. When I run groups I always incorporate some type of art or movement introducing them to more productive coping skills.

I was able to contribute to the field by publishing my first book. It was a compilation of interviews of my pediatric bone marrow transplant patients and their families. They were asked about the process and asked to offer advice to others going needing the same treatment. I was able to distribute it for free across the United States for patients and their families.

My second book was a foundation of my years of creating a cancer young adult support group. It gave social work students a guide to creating groups for their clients. And I was able to record the experiences of my patients to inspire young adults with cancer.

Having this opportunity to be present with some dedicated oncology caregivers is a privilege for me. I have always wanted to ask oncology healthcare providers these questions. Essentially their experience can guide and inspire new clinicians into the field. To understand the depth of impact and meaning in their lives. I also feel making this a foundation to medical care education is relevant to any professional who wants to work with chronically ill clients. To enlighten students on the emotional connection to our work is valuable.

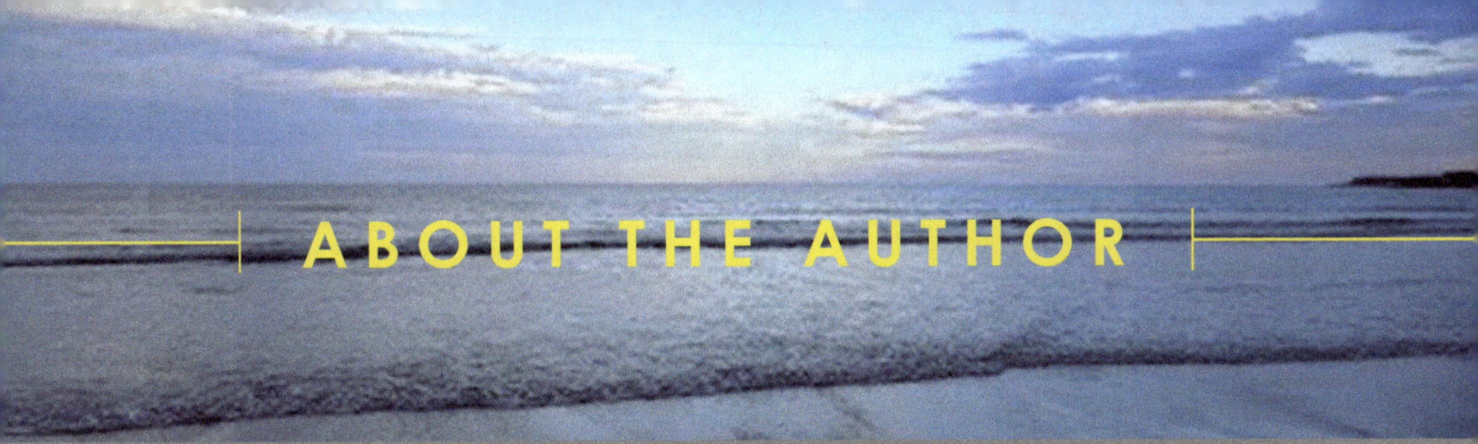

ABOUT THE AUTHOR

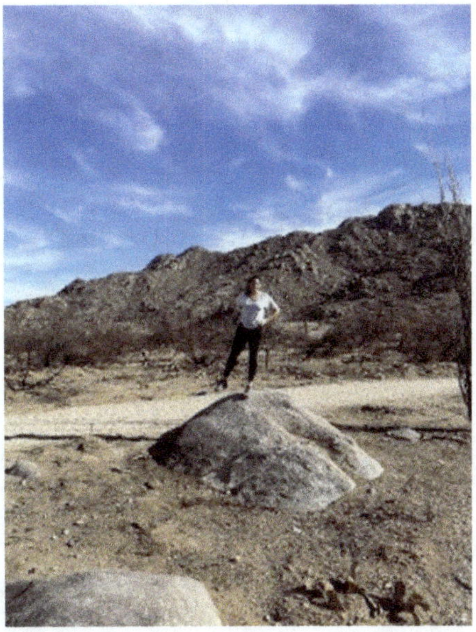

Sarah F. Kurker, MSW, LICSW is an oncology social worker. Her career has included working at University Medical Center, Tucson, Arizona in pediatric bone marrow transplantation (BMT). She also worked at Massachusetts General Hospital in Boston, Massachusetts on the colorectal oncology team. Throughout her career Sarah has created evidence-based group support for oncology patients and their families. She continues to provide this support to young adults with cancer in Tucson, Arizona. Sarah incorporates integrative health into her psychosocial support; including positive self-talk, mindfulness and movement.

She is proud to be a part of published research focusing on grief and loss. Sarah is proud of have been a senior research specialist at the Arizona Cancer Center and completed studies looking at quality of life of cancer patients.

Sarah is a faculty instructor at Arizona State University School of Social Work and Integrative Health Initiative. She has been teaching students for over twenty years connecting clinical work to curriculum. Sarah is passionate about teaching her students self-care in the field.

Sarah's first book publication was distributed through BMT Centers in the United States, free for all families. She interviewed families to get their advice for other's having to go through it. Her second book is a clinical book for social workers on her work with young adults with cancer.

She feels very honored to have supported many going through cancer.

CHAPTER 1

Introduction

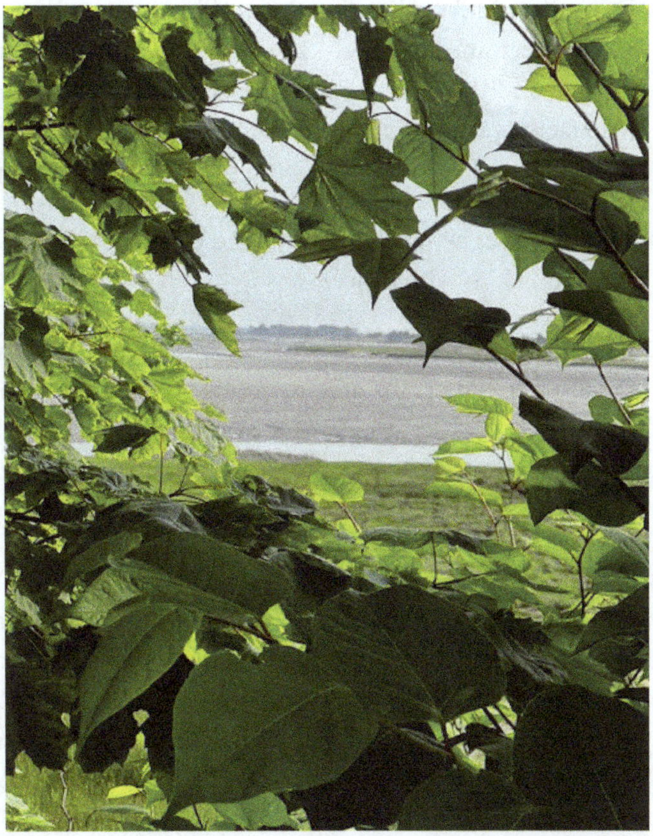

As a senior in high school I had the amazing opportunity to volunteer on 7 East, the in-patient oncology unit at Boston Children's hospital.

When I was in the playroom spending time with a few patients, I was connected, present, and fully mindful of them and my connection. I felt like it was where I should be, the meaning I was meant to do.

Two of my most meaning moments while I volunteered still are prominent in my inspiration of the work I do today. The first meaningful memory was my first memory of mindfulness, making cookies with the kids with cancer in the playroom in a small toaster oven. Each child was hooked up to their chemo and medications, so the poles were prominent in the small room. But the connection of happiness of the moment was profound. Each taking turns putting in ingredients, mixing and talking as we were baking them. It took forever to make maybe a half-dozen cookies, but the feelings of happiness in doing that together gave them a break from the uncontrollable cancer treatment. This activity together gave them hope, peace in the moment, and a time to connect. To bring them those moments made it all worth it. It was the first time I wasn't conscious of time, just was present.

One of my patients, a young girl about 11 years old, was dying. I had played with her over the past months. We spoke different languages, but we always connected. When I came to say my goodbyes, I sat for an endless time, holding her hand and her grandmother's. And I just sat with them. I knew it was what I was gifted to do. I could be present in the hardest moments of life.

At every point of my education, I was able to volunteer with kids with cancer. During my three years at Syracuse University, I was able to volunteer at the oncology outpatient clinic at the local hospital. I connected with some older patients and even got to help plan a holiday party for the kids and their families. I felt so much joy seeing the families be able to be together without the stress of the illness. Giving them those moments felt valuable.

During my MSW education, I was able to research, create, and facilitate a support group for parents with cancer and their kids. It was an amazing 4-week closed group that had interventions for the parents and the kids. I was impressed with the willingness of the radiation oncology therapists to help facilitate it. Seeing the need for support for these parents struggling to get through cancer while parenting and then providing the support had a profound impact on me and the participants.

That semester being on that unit and playing with the kids, I knew I was going to dedicate my career to helping kids with cancer.

Once I began my clinical career, I was touched by each of my pediatric bone marrow transplant (BMT) patients. I was able to create interventions that were thoughtfully individually created to each child. I loved being able to support them on hard days and celebrating our small triumphs together during their inpatient stays that lasted for over a month. Being able to support them through the process everyday for almost 4 months created strong bonds. I think of each of them often, even after all these years.

Then my career took a turn to something new, working in research with adults with cancer. I was able to coordinate recruiting woman with breast cancer for Mindfulness-Based Stress Reduction. I got to know each of these women and heard stories about their life before they were diagnosed with cancer. I was also able to work with another group of women who were in a study comparing walking benefits to NIA (a meditative dance in a group setting). It was fascinating to see this end of the work. It got me thinking about the importance of evidence-based research and intervention in my social work career.

I had an amazing year working at Mass General Hospital (MGH). I was able to be a panel facilitator for Swartz Rounds, talking with my oncology peers about how to work with young adults whom you really connect with. It was an open discussion about boundaries. I ran drop-in support groups for all cancer patients focusing on mindfulness and visualization. I was able work on a team for one doctor for adults with colorectal cancer. It was an amazing feeling to be an integral part of the team; MGH recognized the importance of social work interventions in all their interactions. And I felt that respect. I facilitated a young adult support group that really inspired me to always offer groups to my patients.

I was also able to publish my first book in that year. I had the idea to interview the BMT families that I was the social worker for to ask them about their experience to support others going through it. I unexpectedly learned an immense amount of information about their experience that I only gained in those interviews, despite the fact that I was their social worker. This included patients, sibling, and parents. I am proud to have been able, with the support of some really impactful families in honor of their kids, to distribute this book to all BMT facilities in the United States for free.

An impactful professor and advocate in our social worker profession reached out to ask me to teach at my alma mater. I wasn't sure but wanted to try. I loved being able to inspire other social work students. Connecting my clinical work to curriculum supports my belief in evidence-based practice. Arizona State University (ASU) provides vast opportunities for my growth and development as a faculty instructor. Over the past 20 years of my teaching career, I have been able to develop courses within social work as well as be a part of the Integrative Health Initiative. To be able to teach mindful tools for students in their lives creates such impact. Observing students with stress reduction and personal insight makes me proud on so many levels. And being able to incorporate this in my clinical and teaching skills enhances my impact.

I was able to support my ASU colleague Joanne Cacciatore in her work with grief. I found correlations of grief work and oncology work. Our publication of Sandy Hook Parents broke my heart to transcribe the interviews but gave me honor and a deep appreciation.

I have developed and facilitated a support group for young adults with cancer in Tucson, Arizona. My first clinical created group was at MGH for young adults with cancer, so I had experience. I had wished for a guideline to help create it, but there wasn't a resource available. Therefore, not only did I create this group, but I also wrote a second book on it. Now students in social work have a book they can use when creating groups. What I am most proud of, aside from having the privilege of them trusting in me, was that I recorded their thoughts and was able to have a chapter of their voices and experiences. This is so valuable, and I am proud I was able to publish their voices to support others.

Throughout my years, I have had a great many opportunities to learn from amazing colleagues who inspire me to be creative and continuously improvising in all I do. I find it fascinating when professionals are called to a career in oncology. From my personal impact, I wanted to know what their experience was; maybe to understand my process more. I feel fortunate to be able to have a deep conversation about the impact of caring for patients with cancer.

In the spring of 2024, I was contacted by Kendall Hunt Publishing. A kind thoughtful editor, Hannah, connected, and this book idea was shared. I am thankful she supported this vision.

CHAPTER 2

Sarah F. Kurker, MSW, LICSW

To create the wisdom of oncology healthcare providers, I wanted to create an insightful opportunity to reflect on the participant's career experiences. Developing key questions that provided a meaningful narrative conversation was my goal. I wanted to encompass key components of our work that will inspire new professionals to think about their connection to oncology patients and their families. Below is a list of questions/topics I posed to participants in the semi-structured interviews I conducted and to identify and compile themes and lessons from their answers.

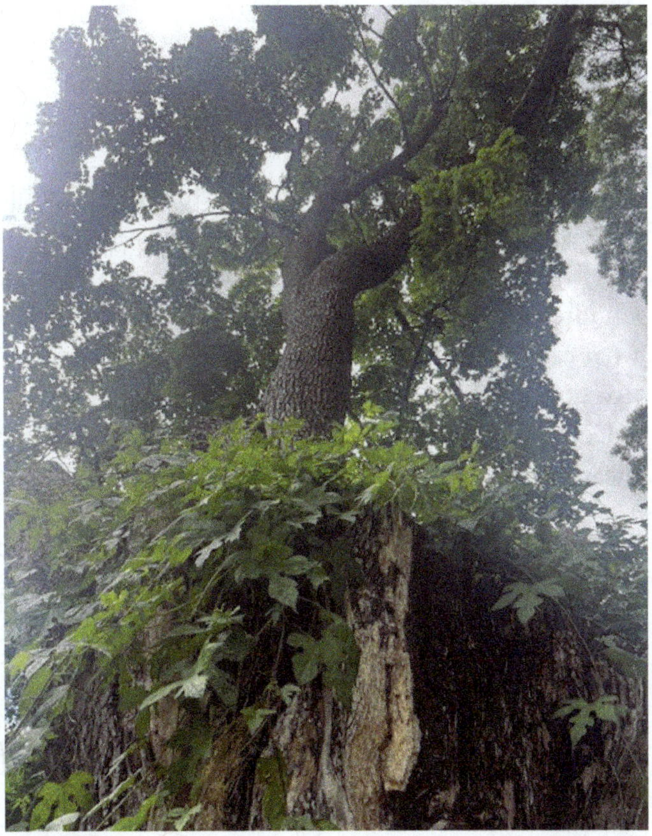

1. Why did you go into oncology?
2. What is your personal meaning from oncology?
3. What insight did you gain from your work?
4. How do you handle the loss, sadness, and grief?
5. Memorable moments to share?
6. What do you do for self-care?
7. Meaning of mindfulness in oncology care?
8. What have you personally brought to oncology care?

9. Wisdom to share to clinicians going into oncology?
10. What does your specific profession bring to patients?
11. How do you rationalize cancer?
12. What has been the most impactful part of your career?
13. Anything else to share?

Follow-up: Anything from our conversation that you want to add or highlight?

I thought incorporating my personal experiences into this format would help me present an overview of the themes I wanted to present and the significance I hope to gain from my colleagues. It also gave me a vision of how I want to facilitate the conversations.

Why Did You Go into Oncology?

I have to say I just had a feeling that this is what would make me happy, and, when I was with kids with cancer, time was irrelevant. I was just present in the moment. On a deeper level, I knew it was my life's calling. As a high school graduate, volunteering with a child life specialist at Boston Children's hospital, I knew I was going to be an oncology healthcare provider. I wasn't quite sure in what capacity I wanted to do so. I was considering a psychiatrist, child life specialist, and maybe a psychologist. I just knew I had to be there for kids with cancer. I would have to say it wasn't so much a decision that I fell compelled to take at that point in my life, but it was more of a realization of my meaning to do so in my lifetime.

Throughout my three years of college, I continued volunteering in different capacities to see where I wanted to make an impact. I found that I liked the social work perspective the most, because I could work with the kids and also their families. I was also part of the oncology medical team, and I was present in the kid's day-to-day experience. I loved that I could integrate me into my interventions, I could play with the kids, and I could support the siblings of the patient. And I could be there for the conversations and treatments. And I would be a part of a team.

What Is Your Personal Meaning from Oncology?

I feel a deep honor from my career. That feeling comes from the patients and families who have trusted me, allowing me to observe and be present in their experience. To this day, I can think of a patient or get a reminder and remember their essence. Being able to be present with people going through cancer, you learn a lot and really connect with them. So, to me, their memory is special because I know I got to be with them during that hard time. I value our connections and the memories.

I feel an abundance of gratitude. After seeing what I have seen in cancer, I know that health is so important. I feel gratitude in all that I do because I have the opportunity. I do things because I know all I have is the now. I believe working in oncology gave me that insight. I have a great appreciation of time. Time is a gift to be present. I know some people don't get time to do the things they want.

I also believe it has made me aware in a way that can cause fear. I was always scared at a cough or at checkups. My choices for health are very prominent since I want to maintain my health. When you hear your patients' stories about their diagnosis, it can bring a fear. I used to have one of the radiation oncologists check my lymph nodes every Friday just to reassure me. To relieve this deep concern, I have to really work on my mind and setting the tone that all is going to be ok. The fear is not rationale but just evolved from the trauma I have witnessed.

From my work with young adults with cancer, I have found a deep appreciation for positive self-talk. I hear these amazing people overcome so much, but then say negative things about themselves. So I focus on this ability to support oneself in my group facilitation, with my students. And I try to use it in my thought process because I think it has such a positive impact on mental health.

What Insight Did You Gain from Your Work?

I have learned that cancer is extremely hard on the patient and all the connections in their life. It impacts physical and emotional development. Cancer's impact is life-long.

I have a connection to a higher being. I feel since I was with many of my patients as they died, I had to make sense of it all. I had to be able to be in the work even in my grief. I actively have to work on my grief. And the grief is different for each patient. To know a patient for months, then going to be there in the middle of the night when they die, then the next day a new patient in the room. That is so hard to process and grieve. How can you be present for your other patients?

Another thing that helped me early in my career was I would have a good fitness routine, getting outside and running before work. Once I started my work, I would dedicate a run to a patient who was struggling. That helped me process and give them good energy in another way.

I learned that no matter the education, the practice of sometimes just being present is enough in this work.

How Do You Handle the Loss, Sadness, and Grief?

As a clinical social worker, I learned that I needed to process closure. The process was different with each patient. Sometimes I would write the family a note; or I would attend a funeral.

I keep the memories close to my heart and remember them a lot. When I think about a patient, I think about the impact they made and the lessons I learned from them.

I try to do a lot of self-care, since early in my career I would get headaches. So, I knew I had to sustain my health to be able to do this longer. And a lot went back to my positive thinking, just reassuring myself I did my best each day and that was enough.

Memorable Moments to Share?

I am definitely thankful that I have years and moments of memories that bring me joy. I could write an entire book and not capture the feelings of moments of each interaction that have impacted me. And some are just too emotional to even put into words.

That being said, here are some that come to mind:

Every Friday I would plan a party at the fish tank. My planning assists were my patients, of course. The children on bone marrow transplant (BMT) were really sick and isolated. This event would give them something to look forward to and a way to see others. I would let them plan an activity. Some would make posters for the weekly event. One-time Marc, a 3-year-old, yelled, “If this is a party, where is the cake?” His mom ran to the cafeteria to get one and from that Friday on we had a cake!

Each patient would impact me, and I always did something just for them. I used to raise money to be able to help with small gifts or gift cards for them to do “normal” things. I always had a craft or toy to play with them if they weren’t up to “social work.” Just being with them and doing something to pass the time made a difference, and I could connect with them in that way.

I really valued our team. I appreciated being part of the oncology team, learning the medical side of cancer, and enhancing my social work interventions to support our client’s best experience. I learned to be an advocate for social work and my families within the team.

One young child would often be alone in the hospital. I would stay if she was throwing up. I would hold the bucket and put my hand on her back. I didn’t want her to be alone.

From every support group I facilitated for patients and for caregivers, I learned an immense amount of the impact of cancer on families. I value that role, and I am happy I put in the effort to have those available to my patients.

What Do You Do for Self-care?

I had always loved movement and being active. I played sports into college. So, movement has always been healing for me. Every morning before work, I would get outside and run. Many runs I would mentally dedicate to one of my patients, knowing they didn't have the privilege to move or be outdoors. It was healing for me to send them good energy when I knew they were really struggling. It was like a form of wishful energy in a prayer. It made me happy to give that dedication.

I love being outdoors and appreciating the nature around me. Being in the moment outdoors, hearing birds, watching clouds, and enjoying the flowers, connects me to a deeper level of meaning. This is my way of small moments of self-care.

While I facilitate my young adult cancer support group, I often will text one of them a beautiful photo of nature and send a quote or a note saying, "Thinking of you," or a note of "You got this." Sometimes I know I can't be there for all their struggles, but it's my way of sending them some hope and care. I do this for anyone in my life who needs some energy—and in terms it makes me thankful I take the time to do it; if I can bring a smile or a reminder to someone, that is beauty in itself. An aspect of this action I do comes from my knowledge that time is not promised, and I know in one breath everything can change. So, if someone comes into my mind, I share it. I do this a lot for the families who have lost a child. If I think of them, I let the families know. To keep their loved one's spirit brings them joy. It is part of my gratitude of being with them in a hard time and honoring who they are.

For each patient who has died, I try to do some sort of closure. It can be a phone call to the parent, a card, or attending a funeral. Sometimes, it's a few things or just one. But I become mindful of the person and my grief for them, and I find a way to honor that. Listening to my emotions about my loss is key to finding out what I need to do to move on, for me, and to gift to the family.

For me, self-care is a mindset—constantly encouraging myself and reminding myself I am doing enough. Throughout my career, I would feel sad and guilty for not doing enough for a patient. So I had to shift my thoughts into I did what I could and to the best of my ability.

I have a strong spiritual faith that supports me through this work.

Meaning of Mindfulness in Oncology Care?

I do believe that my meaning in life, becoming an oncology social worker, grew from my mindful connection. I feel present and, in the moment, when I am with patients. I am aware of them and my connection to them and that mindful connection allows me to do the work I do. As I learn from social work I meet the client where they are at, the essence of being mindful, and I resonate with that in my work. I feel in especially hard times, facing death, I know just being present for them is all I can do to help.

What Have You Personally Brought to Oncology Care?

In my first job after getting my MSW, I incorporated parties for the kids. It always made them happy, and for them it was something to look forward to. I really liked giving gifts. I would donate my time and money and then get the kid's personal gifts. They never knew it was from me but that it was just donated. And to complete this, I also had to learn how to write grants to get funding for things for my patients' families. I feel that not only did it support my families, but that it also created awareness in the community about what these kids go through. Sometimes within grant writing I would get to connect with amazing people in the community who wanted to do more to support our patients. This grant writing and community collaboration would be a foundation of the work I did throughout my career.

As an MSW intern, I was always aware of themes within my clients. If there was a need that was not being met, I would create a way to fulfill it. Many times, that came in the form of support groups. At the Arizona Cancer Center, I created one for caregivers. And I learned they just needed to be heard and not have as much structure. At Mass General Hospital, my team had so many young adults, so I created a young adult support group.

With my love for mindfulness and movement, I started taking my sessions outdoors. I would ask parents if they wanted to move while we caught up. I felt that was a way for them to benefit from nature and moving their bodies. I called it a walk-and-talk.

Over the past few years, I have really been able to incorporate my photography of nature into supporting not only patients but also colleagues—sending them a quick note and photo letting them know I am thinking about them, or something I appreciate about them.

I also think about my integration of teaching students at Arizona State University and being able to share clinical foundations from my work. Presenting at conferences and publishing research I have participated in create a macro-level influence that I always feel is important to me.

Wisdom to Share to Clinicians Going into Oncology?

I would say to find supports within your career that can support you. Having a mentor who you can debrief with is a great way to continue your growth and development. Mentors can be within your profession or others within oncology.

Be flexible in your self-care; it may change along the path of your professional development or as you get into new roles. Creating your self-care is ever-changing and ever-evolving, which may entail engaging deeply with the process of raising your own awareness of what you need to do to care for yourself in this emotionally draining work.

Deeply listen to your patients and integrate their experience into your work.

What Does Your Specific Profession Bring to Patients?

The beauty of social work is that you can be with patients in their everyday experience fighting cancer. I also like to be a part of the medical team, advocating for your clients' psychosocial care. Within social work, you can make an impact on so many levels. On the micro-level lecture, you can provide interventions that help each client. Then you can impact the mezzo and macro by establishing program and support groups and even changing policy. This is really the beauty of social work.

How Do You Rationalize Cancer?

I struggle with this all the time. It just doesn't make sense or have a reason why kids get cancer, or anyone. I think I have had to process that bad things happen for no reason. That being said, having my faith helps me.

What Has Been the Most Impactful Part of Your Career?

Having the true honor of getting to know each of my patients and learning from them has been the most impactful part of my career.

Publishing my books on pediatric BMT and young adult support groups feels like an impact for those who read it and learn from it. This experience of my vision and interviews and sharing it with new oncology professionals is significant.

I really value my teaching career at Arizona State University, and inspiring my students makes me proud. That being said, what I have learned from students inspires me to keep growing and learning always.

CHAPTER 3

Terry Shapiro: Oncology Nurse Practitioner

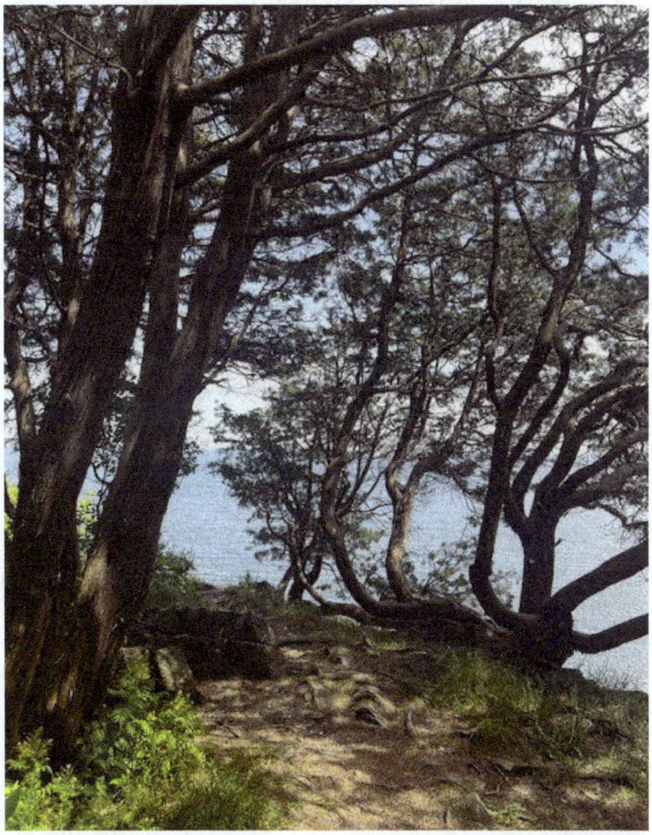

When I first met Terry, I felt her energy that illuminated confidence. When she was with our team or with the families of patients, her voice was heard. She was able to connect with the families in a profound way; getting to know them and making the interactions personal. It was my first MSW job when I worked with Terry. Her presence taught me a lot about how to be part of the oncology team and find my role. I remember being in awe of her clinical decisions and how she would explain them to the families. I was also impressed that she wrote a clinical book on bone marrow transplantation (BMT) protocols. Of course, I still value my signed copy. Although we only worked together for a little over two years, we have always kept in touch when she comes to town for a visit. I was excited to have this opportunity to ask her these questions for the first time in all of the years we have known each other. She has recently retired, so I was thankful for this opportunity to have a deep conversation.

Why Did You Go into Oncology?

For Terry, the field of oncology came to her. As a new graduate nurse she took her first job at Shands Teaching Hospital at the University of Florida where she was given multiple choices of which specialty care unit she wanted to work. She was intrigued by oncology, and Shands was only the fifth hospital in the United States to open a BMT unit. BMT is often referred to as "cancer's boot camp." Terry wanted the challenge of "new and daring" for her first job. She was a young adult at the age of just 22, and most of her early patients died from the actual treatment of BMT itself. However, from the start she knew she had to stay in this extremely challenging work, and would often think, "If I don't care for these poor patients, who will take care of them?" She recognized at this very early stage in her career that when patients who come to BMT, it's their only option for survival. That honor of being there for them has stayed with her throughout her career. She recognized early that BMT is the bootcamp of oncology treatments; intense, and she never gave up on trying to save her patients.

> *In my early 20s, I refused to give up on them like, who's going to take care of them if it's not me? Who is going to take care of these people at this horrible juncture in their life, I mean, a cancer diagnosis is devastating for anyone. But given how young these people were, and how vulnerable they were. And how little was left for them. At the time, only me and a handful of nurses and physicians just kind of stuck with it. And then it was so incredible to be a part of a treatment modality where we were learning so much at such a rapid rate. There's still a number of patients who still do not survive even now, but we are now cure a majority of patients. And so that evolution has been incredible … and it's also been so cool to be a part of a high-risk situation where we were learning so much.*

So even when others would suggest she do another type of work, she knew she needed to stay with oncology. She shared about the medical progression and how the BMT care has changed over the years. We are not just "trying" to save them; we are also trying to better understand the many complex complications that are associated with BMT.

What Is Your Personal Meaning from Oncology?

Terry talks about her "big saves" and making her patients smile by being funny on morning rounds. She is proud of the energy she was able to give them during a really difficult time in their lives. Those connections gave her meaning every day. To my surprise, our conversation wasn't much about the medical decisions she made but the connections she made with her patients. A deep, meaningful connection. She talks about brightening their day, each one individually.

She also talks about the medical impact and that she has "seen it all." When her career brought her to Hershey, Pennsylvania, to help manage their new pediatric BMT unit at Penn State Medical Center, she was a leader in the field. She was able to teach her team about things that she had medically experienced with her clients over the years.

In the early years, patients who needed a bone marrow transplant didn't survive, but that changed over the many years, and now we have learned how to get them through this tough therapy in order to cure their cancer. It really became like a huge challenge for me. You know, the rarer the complication, the more interesting it became at that point. I've probably seen just about everything in the field after doing this almost 40 years. Everything. There were physicians and nurses new to the field that were just marveled by my knowledge and experience, like, "Oh, God! How did you know that?" "Because I've done it."

What Insight Did You Gain from Your Work?

Terry expressed being emotional and human in this work. She stated that this approach was more important in the field of oncology than being strong and "put together' in the difficult situations like when a patient dies or experiences treatment failures such as relapse of their cancer. Terry spoke about being able to show her emotions when working with patients' families in difficult situations.

Terry recently retired after 40 years of caring for both adult and mostly pediatric oncology patients. She shared about how families continue to contact her. How they have expressed their gratitude for her impact on their lives. And that meaning is a tribute to her career.

and just said what a big difference I made in their lives, and how they always appreciated me caring for their child or loved one ....

How I could actually make their kid or their family member, you know, smile, but at the same time not undermine the significance and the seriousness of the situation. I think, also being able to emphasize and say I was never a stoic clinician. And I think a lot of people who chose oncology are like this; somewhat afraid to show their emotions to patients and their families.

I mean I've laughed, I've cried, and I never felt like that was crossing any kind of boundary. If you're at the bedside of a dying child's and you're weeping with the parents, I think actually, I've found that approach to be a lot more therapeutic than just trying to stand tall and be strong.

Another concept that Terry shared is how much she loves being able to follow her oncology patients and their families throughout their lifetimes. That connection of knowing families and kids for their entire life is profound. So, her work is impacted through all their life stages; through rigorous treatment and then their attempt at "normalcy" again.

Memorable Moments to Share?

Terry conveyed how amazing it feels when some of our mutual patients have significant life milestones, like getting married or having a child. And that intoxicating feeling that I have been some part of it … that it "feels so good."

This young lady was 13, and just had this effervescent personality, and of course she had a horrible diagnosis. She had Ewing's sarcoma, and then she developed myelodysplasia (treatment-related leukemia) as a result of her Ewing's sarcoma therapy. Her stem cell donor search was not great, so she had to have an unrelated, partially mismatch, transplant which is super risky, but she had no other choice if she was going to survive. She had a complicated transplant and then she relapsed early on after her transplant, and then also had a life-threatening viral infection. Yes, she just had one of those transplants that was just one complication after another. She suffered greatly. Her mother was by far one of the most highly evolved parents I've ever cared for. She was amazing. And I was pretty tight with the mother and her child as well. Since she had such a difficult course, she had been in the hospital for more than 3 months since she was suffering from multiple, life threatening complications. We were able to get her leukemia back in remission with a risky, donor lymphocyte infusion. Unfortunately, she was also suffering not only the life-threatening viral infection, but also had really severe, multisystem graft-versus-host disease.

After being able to get her back into remission, I felt like we were starting to turn things around, but her adenovirus infection was worsening. At that point we got pediatric palliative care involved, but continued to treat her virus aggressively. These days we try to get them involved much earlier than we used to as an added layer of support for the child and the family. But anyway, I was rounding on her one morning and Mom looked at me and said, "You know what you know on paper." I was being somewhat encouraging and saying, "oh, this is better, that is better." I'm a very much an intuitive clinician, but at the same time, can keep things real. I knew my girl was extremely ill, and I don't think I was not in denial at the time, but her mother looked at me, and she says, "You know what? My daughter, my beautiful daughter, has not smiled at me in over a month, and I think she's suffering severely. So, you know, I think it's time here." And I was like "What? I'm not ready. Wow, I'm not, I'm not ready." And it was the first time in my entire career that I had ever felt that way .... You know, where the parent was ready for their child to die, and I was not ... actually, giving me a huge reality check. You truly learn something about yourself from every person (and their family) that you care for.

Terry talks about patients' families reaching out to her when she retired, even families of children who had died. The feeling of gratitude from these families is truly what kept her going all of these years. This is why she remained in oncology for her entire career. Terry shares she has "endless amounts of connections," seeing families every day and many times a day during this incredibly hard time. I really connect with that and know for oncology clinicians that really sums it up wholeheartedly.

What Do You Do for Self-care?

Although we didn't talk specifically about this, Terry shared she never had time in her career for self-care. She started in this intense field as a very young adult with passion and a strong sense of challenge. She then became a mom and had to dedicate all her non-work time to her two girls as she provided consistent, personal care for her oncology patients. She shared that she would often be with her kids at a party or event and then had to leave to return to the hospital to see a patient. She reports that her thoughts were often consumed with thinking about her patients and how best to treat them.

And now that she has retired she is finally doing her self-care, traveling and having fun!

Meaning of Mindfulness in Oncology Care?

Terry was mindful throughout her career by connecting with her patients and really being there for them. Making them smile in the moments.

What Have You Personally Brought to Oncology Care?

Terry brought her diligence, intelligence, and extreme empathy in caring for her patients. Terry's intrinsic presence is evident in every interaction.

Wisdom to Share to Clinicians Going into Oncology?

Terry talks about how difficult and overwhelming it can be to take care of kids with cancer. And its not for everyone. But finding the true meaning in all the work really helps.

How Does She Rationalize Cancer?

Given her recent retirement, Terry has time reflect on this. She feels it comes down to the fact that "bad shit just happens to all people," and that includes good people and children and young people. Working in this field has made it challenging for her to connect to a religion, including believing in a higher power that would allow the suffering of children, or anyone for that matter. She overcomes this challenge by acknowledging her strong belief that she has to be there for those suffering since there are few clinicians who feel they can. She feels Oncology is "a calling"; a profession that gives you deep meaning and a profession where one can truly really make an impact—the deep meaning that you can only explain by being with patients and their families facing cancer.

> *So, twice in my career things occurred that defy logical explanation to me. I'm not a particularly religious person, but you know I do have a good level of spirituality. I recognize there are things that happen that we can't explain. The first one involves a little girl named Kiley, who was 7 and also not a great situation since she suffered from both pulmonary Adenovirus and relapse of her leukemia. Kiley was smart, sweet, kind, and very charismatic. You couldn't help but be drawn to her. Kiley was clearly not going to survive despite our most heroic efforts. Her mother felt passionately that she did not want Kiley to die in the hospital. She wanted her to be at home, in her bed, with her dog, surrounded by the people she loves. Terry reluctantly agreed and expressed to the mother that it would be a challenge to manage Kiley at home, but exclaimed "OK, then that's what we're going to do." Terry reported that kids who are dying of pulmonary problems are the hardest to manage at home on hospice because of air hunger and extreme discomfort. It's really a hard symptom for hospice and parents of the dying person to actually have to manage. The visible suffering is a hard thing to watch. Given the fatal nature of her disease, both Kiley and her mother felt very strongly that she needed to be home. This little girl was "magical" and so highly evolved given the situation of her impending death. And she said, "Mommy, I do want to be at home. It will be alright, mommy." At this point, Terry felt that Kiley would probably only survive a few days at home before needing to return to the hospital for management of her air hunger and pain. It was time to mobilize our forces to try to make her desire to die at home a reality. Before she*

left the hospital, Kiley expressed to her mother that there were a number of things she wanted to do before she died. Things like she wanted to pet an alligator. She wanted to meet Taylor Swift. She was dying around Christmas time, so she also wanted to have Christmas carolers sing to her.

Kiley's mom moved quickly on social media posting a list of her daughter's last wishes as "Kiley's bucket list." Kiley was dying almost 10 years ago, so at the time, the popularity of social media was just beginning to explode. Mom's post went viral within 24 hours of her leaving the hospital to die at home. In the meantime, we were working hard with hospice to get her home on morphine and oxygen while her story was going viral on social media. It was an incredible thing to watch and be a part of. Hershey has this small zoo named "Zoo America," so they call in the midst of trying to get her home, and within a few hours, they bring this little alligator up to the hospital so Delaney could pet the alligator! In the same day, someone contacted Taylor Swift who was in Australia at the time, but she freaking face-timed her the first night she was home on Hospice!

We were able to get her home, I think, like 2 days before Christmas. The story of her bucket list was in the news. The family lived in this little town near Reading, PA, and on her first night at home, 3,000 people from their small town showed up on her doorstep to sing Christmas Carols as Kiley listened and smiled ear to ear from her bedroom window. In the midst of fulfilling Kiley's bucket list, I had to see her in our clinic on Christmas Eve just to make sure she was tucked in with transfusions, and to assure that her oxygen and pain management were sufficient at home. Since she was medically fragile, she was transported to clinic that day via ambulance. When she arrived in clinic, she was visibly air hungry and highly uncomfortable. Both she and her family appeared incredibly stressed.

When she arrived at my clinic, and I said, somewhat exasperated to her mother, "How long she been like this?" She was visibly suffering, which was not okay, like I can't tolerate watching a child suffer, no matter how badly she yearns to be at home. I was close to tears and both Kiley and her mother could sense how upset I was. I told her mother that she can't be at home this air hungry and uncomfortable, and her mom exclaimed, "You've got 8 hours to work your magic because my child does not want to die here. You've got 8 hours to like work your magic, Terry." So, I quickly admitted her, got her switched over to a Fentanyl drip, jacked up her oxygen, and I sent her back home. It was, after all Christmas Eve. No small miracle in and of itself. I stayed with Kiley and her family until they left that night. I remember giving both mom and Kiley the biggest hug imaginable ... and yet I wondered if this was the right call.

Later that night, Abby (my daughter) who was a Freshman in high school at the time asked me to sleep with her in her bed. Until she was 8 years old, Abby was always my kid that would creep into my bed at night; nearly every night. It had been years since I slept it with Abby, but on that Christmas Eve, she asked me to sleep with her. Given the explosion of "Kiley's Bucket List" on social media both of my daughters and all of their friends were following Kiley's story closely on social media. Earlier in the evening, I had shared with Abby how hard my day had been without going into great detail. Given the difficulty of my day, I welcomed her invitation. Abby's bed is wedged under a large window in her bedroom. The head of her bed is basically the window.

When I had gone to bed with Abby that night, my last thought was of Kiley. Was it the right thing to send her back home the day before? I was like, "God, I hope that was the right thing." Blah blah blah, but took comfort in her mom's saying, "Look! She's … she seems to be in a better place on the Fentanyl" I fell asleep wondering if I should have just kept her in the hospital to manage her comfort until she drew her last breath.

At 4:18 on Christmas morning, I woke up with a really sharp pain in my stomach, which was unusual for me.

I sat up, and Abby's awoke and asked, "Mommy, are you okay?" I told her "I'm okay." And then I laid back down and I looked out of the window, and a huge Shooting Star soared through the night sky. I said to Abby, "I think Kiley just died." Abby picked up her phone and reported that no one had posted anything, including her mom. I asked Abby what time it was, and she reported that it was 4:18 AM. We then fell back to sleep. At 8 AM, Abby woke me to tell me that Kiley's mom had just posted on social media that Kiley had died that Christmas morning at 4:18 AM, the exact moment I saw that shooting star. I think that was Kiley's way of telling me that I had done the right thing getting her home to her bed, with her dog, surrounded by the people who loved her. She was telling me she was ok.

Terry recalls the second time she had an intense spiritual experience involving a child she was close to:

It was right before Thanksgiving, and I was standing across the bed from the father of a sweet girl that was also dying. Chloe was 15 and was deteriorating from an overwhelming cytomegalovirus infection. Her dad, in fact, contacted me recently on Facebook, to tell me he still thinks frequently about this shared spiritual experience.

I was leaving later in the day for Thanksgiving in Connecticut. I explained to dad and Chloe that I just wanted to make sure they were tucked in before I left. Chloe appeared asleep though our entire interaction. It was early in the morning before the sun had come up and her room was almost completely dark. As I was explaining Chloe's deterioration to her dad, a huge flash of light bolted across her bed. I looked pensively at her dad and said, "Did you see that?" To which he reluctantly answered, "Yeah, I saw it .... I was hoping you would say that you saw it too." Chloe was on a cardiac monitor and was also connected to multiple IV pumps, so I dispelled the flash of light as some sort of electric event and reported to the dad that I would have the nurse call Clinical Engineering to come and evaluate her equipment.

Chloe died the following day while I was away for Thanksgiving. A few days after her funeral, her father came to visit the hospital. He shared with me that the day after she died, he went into her bedroom at home and curled up in her bed and wrapped his arms around her pillow. Chloe had a full-length mirror in her teenage girl room that was turned toward the hallway. As dad was looking in the mirror and thinking about her, he said he saw that same light in the reflection of the mirror that we both saw the day before she died. He needed to know once again, that I had also seen it.

CHAPTER 4

Marsha Drozdoff

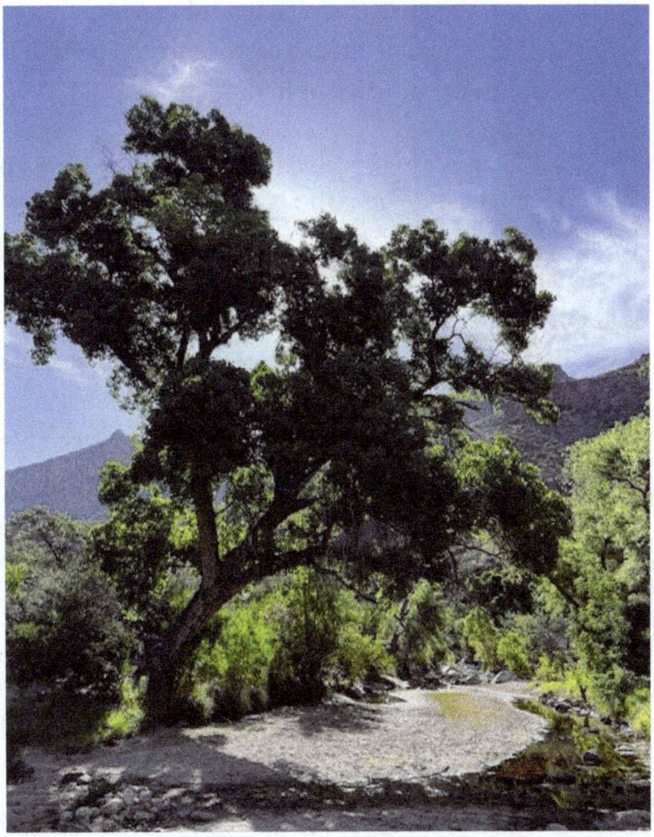

I feel fortunate to have had Marsha be my social work supervisor at the Arizona Cancer Center as a second-year intern when I was attending Arizona State University social work program. Marsha dedicated some of her time to support students who were getting their internship. I learned so many valuable lessons from her. The most profound was to just be available to patients and know *that* the ones who need you will come to you. I was so eager to meet all patients and would get disappointed when it didn't go as planned. But resetting my mindset that it will all work out each day to see *who* I am supposed to see was such a positive change for me. That view has helped me *throughout* my career. And in oncology, it's *particularly* important because with all the trauma that patients go through sometimes you *may* spend all day with a patient and their family, and that is ok. Marsha knew this skill and was able to pass it onto me. The foundation of this skill is mindfulness; being present with *whom* you are *with*, instead of thinking about all that needs to be done.

Marsha was influential in the radiation oncology team. She was able to educate all on the importance of social work interventions, self-care, and integrative support. When I first started, I was receiving so many referrals because they knew the importance of our work in their patients' lives.

Marsha's talents in social work were really evident in her facilitation of support groups. She developed and facilitated a very impactful support group for woman with breast cancer. These women were dedicated to the process of group and to supporting each other. In observing the keen skills of making everyone feel valued and heard, Marsha inspired me to facilitate groups during my career. I was fortunate during my internship to be able to participate in Marsha's group and to fill in when she was away.

Spending any time with Marsha made it evident that she is centered and mindful. She has the ability to intrinsically validate other's experiences. I believe this stems from her own connection to mindfulness and to her practice of Reiki.

I am so grateful to Marsha for her impact on one of my favorite patients, Robby. He was an insightful, charismatic little one who had cancer since he was under the age of 2. Despite this, Robby loved life and every moment in it. He was getting some treatment in radiation oncology, and Marsha immediately connected to him. She offered him an opportunity to be videotaped to inspire other kids going through cancer. Robby was always willing to support others, despite his struggle with cancer. I was able to observe the video project, and Marsha was able to validate his life and its meaning. And for a 10-year-old to have this chance to share his story and meaning was profound. I am thankful for her giving him this chance; it's such an honor to his life. To this day I use this video with my students because Robby shared the essence of visualization and how it helped him fight cancer. To this day I miss Robby and hold his being in my heart. Marsha's creative and out-of-the-box intervention provided such an impact to his life. He was able to thank his grandmother for being there for him; when no one believed he couldn't walk, she would carry him.

And to know that Marsha had that same life-changing impact on her other patients throughout her career inspires me to be creative in the way that I connect to my patients.

Why Did You Go into Oncology?

As a young college student, Marsha overheard someone talking at a phone booth about social work. At Brooklyn College, Marsha was indecisive about how she could best professionally impact others. Clinical psychology seemed like the right direction. In speaking with this stranger, however, she was encouraged to go into social work because of the additional benefit of starting an internship right away.

Marsha just knew she wanted to help people and felt drawn to working in a medical setting. Her second-year internship was at Downstate Medical Center where she happened to be assigned to OB/GYN oncology. And although she didn't actually choose oncology, it felt like an excellent fit and provided a deep sense of purpose.

> *There was something about oncology. It was where I started growing, and where I continued to work after my internship. It was a really rich experience.*

As a young adult, Marsha worked with an oncologist who had high expectations. She had to present the psychosocial situation of all the patients each week. She learned her voice and how to communicate the social work perspective. She was able to be an advocate for her patients throughout their journey and process of cancer. She talks about working with a patient for whom she had to reset the acceptance of blood transfusions to save her life. The client initially thought the blood was from animals, which was against her values. Marsha had to communicate these issues to the oncology team for them to better educate her and address her fears.

Marsha shares about the generational impact of her work. She said early on they didn't discuss the topics of death or dying with patients, even though their patients were facing death. And then Dr. Kubler Ross published his work on death and dying that began to change the conversation and, consequently, how she interacted with patients and families throughout her career.

> *And so it was like learning that there's so much to do in oncology that people were not doing (talking about death).*
>
> *I couldn't change people from dying, but I could change their experience of living with very serious disease with dying being part of that.*

When asked to create a support group, Marsha intrinsically asked her patients about the best way to get patients to attend. They said to make it fun and social. So, her first group was based on bingo and sharing time together! She remembers one young woman who she attended and was facing death. The group was the motivation for that young woman to get dressed up, put on makeup, leave the hospital room, and connect with others.

Marsha shares how she was creative in her social work support.

> *We had a young girl who was, I think, about 16 and in high school; she was going to die, and she wasn't going to make it even to her graduation. She probably was not getting out*

of the hospital except on very brief passes. I questioned what could I do from a social work perspective? What was important to her from her developmental stage? What could we do? Where is the hope? I couldn't change her prognosis, but I could help make changes in her life so that her family could perceive her in a different way of celebrating her, not just mourning her. I decided to work with her principal and explored what we could do to get her graduated, earlier. She was still trying to do some of her school work in the hospital. We knew it didn't look good. We all (the oncology team) chipped in for her senior ring. I think we got some kind of music in.

Her principal and a teacher came up. And we graduated her and took photos. We celebrated her milestone. And then she didn't die. She didn't die yet. So, the next question was what do we do now? Where is the next goal? Because that's what social work can do, helping our clients with setting and achieving goals. What could we do to help her stay engaged in life. And so, I talked to her oncologist and I explained this. I said, look, "She's alive. What are we going to do with her?" We looked for a solution together. She had taken secretarial skills. I said, "Don't you have any work she could do in the hospital?" That was the day of typewriters, and they would bring up a typewriter to her room. He would give her some reports that weren't confidential. And she would type for him, got paid, and meaning. She was engaged in meaning and worth every day in her life until the end.

This experience exemplifies how Marsha, early in her career, was able to intervene with a hopeful orientation for her patients. She brought community and meaning to her patients and that in turn provided them with hope. This definitely helped many to transition easier and perhaps more at peace.

Marsha explains that she never experienced burnout, even though it was statistically documented to be high in both social work and oncology. She attributes this to her dedication to meditation, creating value and meaning. Due to her connection to Buddhism, she sets intensions each day on how she can be the most present with her patients and to bring the best essence of herself to work.

How can I manifest what I'm supposed to be doing today and to being open and receptive to that learning. And the other part that's very Buddhistic is what we call "faith equals daily life." It was always about what we call doing one's human revolution. What am I going to do to grow today? What are the possibilities? How can I change and transform this situation? What can I do to keep improving while finding the personal meaning within each challenge?

What Is Your Personal Meaning from Oncology?

Marsha gained deep insights from her work in oncology all these years. She was able to retire a few years back, but her stories and impact are all very tangible now. If you didn't know, you would think she is still doing the work. So, the long-term impact is meaningful.

> *My patients were my best teachers, and I was so privileged that they were so kind, and trusted me while teaching me so much about life; there is so much value within our lives no matter what.*

Marsha was able to really learn from each of her patients. She values the oncology caregiving setting and believes some of these lessons would only happen with patients facing cancer.

> *This is very, very real, very poignant. Though not always easy. Obviously, you learn a lot through what we experience in people's deep suffering. It was a continuous process. It's really about our humanness and what we all share together.*

I think it helps you to live better. Because you realize that it could be any one of us. It's not like a depressed state where you might think: "Oh, I'm going to die today or tomorrow," but it's more about what is a greater appreciation of our lives and what is important now. We know that's not being in denial. There's not saying: "Okay, if I go to all the doctors and do everything for wellness, it's not going to happen to me." We see people in their teens or twenties, and you can't explain why they have a cancer and may die so early in their lives. There's no right justification for why or how?

How Do You Handle the Loss, Sadness, and Grief?

Marsha discovered hope and healing through the losses. This perspective helped her to balance the hard times of the work that oncology healthcare professionals do.

Memorable Moments to Share

Marsha shared a story of a young patient about 16. She was dying, and Marsha spent extra time after work being with her mom. The doctor had predicted she would die by a certain day, and yet this patient lived days past that time. It was like she was determined to have some control in the situation; she wanted to go in a way that was on her terms.

And we're telling her (the patient) how close she is. And we're cheering her on as if she's doing a marathon. And sure enough. Not only did she make it past that day. She went one extra day just to make sure. So, sadness? Sure. But also victories and reframed successes.

What Do You Do for Self-care?

Marsha has a solid foundation in self-care. With her connection to Buddhism and her practice of meditation, these would center her. In addition, she was able to appreciate nature and get outdoors.

It's a multitude of things. One is, of course, you know, having a daily practice; I always say to people, they don't have to be chanting, do yoga or use alternative modalities, but find something that helps you to refresh and renew yourself. For me, It was also getting outside in nature.

During difficult and overwhelming times, I think the mantra that I used the most was: "You can't be all things to all people, at all times." I could only do my very best. I could give my heart and try to identify additional resources or ideas. I did meditate about my clients and their welfare while also taking care of myself in the process.

This is such a valiant point, because it is a process to get into this mindset. And it really connects to the one she taught me as an intern. It also connects to positive psychology where you know you are doing the best you possibly can, and, importantly, you are meeting people where they are at.

Marsha also shares that having a pet, a dog that made her smile, brought a lot of joy for her. This connection to animals is so profound that in her retirement she volunteers with homeless pets awaiting adoption. She is still giving of herself and receiving that feeling of joy from bringing healing to others. Even furry babies.

Early on, Marsha heard from a colleague that it gets easier over time and that you stop feeling sad. But Marsha felt that as a clinician you really do have to feel the experience and the emotions that go along with that. She was able to practice Reiki for her own healing, wellness, and self-care even on a difficult day; she was also able to incorporate this into her care for patients which soothed her own heart in being able to offer this additional comfort and care to her patients in need.

Meaning of Mindfulness in Oncology Care?

Marsha had the vision of hope in all her interactions with patients and families. That centering of hope, and finding opportunity in her work, was a strong foundation of care. This in itself is mindfulness. Being present for people to find their hope throughout the living or dying processes.

> *Where do you find the hope in the situation? And how and where do you help your clients to find this hope as well. So, as we know in oncology, even if it looks like there's difficult circumstances and a poor prognosis, could the hope be that someone could be made more comfortable, or that they stay alive for a family member to arrive or better prepare for the loss? What was so profound in dealing with grief and loss was, identifying what I could do to help someone; the whole essence of healing is that we all have something to heal within our lives and supporting that intention is what we can do best.*

Throughout our conversation for this book, Marsha shares about hope and healing and how it was significant in her work. Having that mindset of hope and healing changes the perspective from cancer and death to celebrating life, each and every day and each and every second of it.

What Have You Personally Brought to Oncology Care?

> *And I think back to one of my clients, a really beautiful woman. She was about 82 and very elegant and tall. She had colorectal cancer, I believe, and was on chemotherapy and doing radiation treatments; she'd always come into her sessions wearing a hat and not a sun type hat. She was classy, and she also wore gloves. She requested Reiki from me. That was one of the modalities I could offer to patients for stress reduction, relaxation, and to support symptom management. And during this time, I was also involved in an art and healing program; it came up during our conversation, and I asked her whether she would please consider taking one of the classes. She's had said this wasn't for her. She, however, agreed to try just one session; she loved it and participated in the whole series while also receiving Reiki from me. What happens with Reiki is that the energy can help to release blocked emotions. Our bodies and minds contain the narrative of our lives on a cellular level. And as the energy flows, it helps memories to gently, comfortably, effortlessly come to the surface so one could take a peek or more if one chooses to, which in her case she did.*
>
> *She had unfortunately had the experience of 2 of her children drowning. One was a very young boy in a swimming pool in a summer program, and the other was a daughter in her*

twenties. I was so moved and impacted by these traumas in her life. Yet, here's this woman who appears so well-put-together. It became apparent, however, that these were two areas of grief and loss that had not been resolved; some of that came up during our Reiki sessions, and I truly believe there was tremendous healing as shown in her paintings from the art and healing program. One exercise was supposed to be the integration of one's life. She painted 82 circles with the most gorgeous colors. Only 2 circles had light gray in it. It's like the grief and loss which could have overflowed with darkness instead had found its place; her life as a whole was still beautiful and rich: Grief and loss could be balanced with hope and healing even in the face of her own impending death.

Marsha was able to implement program development in her work. She would listen deeply to her patients and create programs that would support them. The following remembrance shares so many elements of this. Once Marsha started observing the benefits from receiving Reiki treatments for herself and took trainings and initiated a Reiki practice, she knew she needed to offer this for her patients. She took a strategic process by teaching it first to her coworkers so they knew the benefits for their patients. Marsha eventually got a space in radiation oncology to provide the Reiki to patients, families, and even staff. And if you look at the progression of integrative health in oncology, Marsha was influential in getting this to Arizona patients.

In sharing about this fabulous woman and how she helped to create and implement various programs such as the Arts and Healing program, music for recovery and congruence for women with breast cancer, Reiki classes, and more, these programs were only available due to Marsha's hard work. She would develop the programs and get funding to support them. This is a profound legacy of care.

Personally, I took a Reiki class to learn to work on myself because my former Reiki Master Teacher said there was much to work on, and it would be better to do it daily. And then what happened is that as I started getting better, it became ethically impossible not to offer it to my clients and integrate it into my clinical practice, because I would see patients lying there hurting physically and emotionally. I remember seeing a patient on a stretcher waiting for a test, and I don't know why they couldn't give him pain medication, but he was in so much pain, physical pain. And I asked him, "Can I put my hands on you?" "I'm doing this healing modality called Reiki. It might quiet some of your distress," and he said, "please," and it quieted his system. He soon drifted into a restful sleep.

I had a little one, a 3-year-old, who spent most of her life in the hospital with neuroblastoma or something. She had a big tumor under her neck. She had the most beautiful and soulful eyes. I didn't get to ask the family, "Can I do Reiki?" Because I didn't plan to. The little one was crying from pain, and she took my hand to where it hurt; within minutes she fell asleep.

So as these experiences kept occurring, I started getting intrigued. It's like spirit, or energy, or perhaps the divine, whatever you want to call it, kept saying to me, "You need to do this." It was not a conscious decision initially; I would just refer patients to people in the community for Reiki. And then I discussed it with my manager. I knew most of all I needed my oncology team to better know about Reiki. I knew that if I was going to try to introduce it, the doctors, nurses, and therapists needed to get comfortable with this as an intervention. So, I offered the whole team, a taste of Reiki and to come to my office during a break possibly for 10 minutes; some doctors actually came in during their lunch hour, and they would give someone else their beeper not to be disturbed. Not everyone did it, but those that did were impressed. It started to change the culture of what Social Work could offer to their patients. My team felt that not only do they know Marsha, and trust her, because whatever she does she does with integrity, but that this is something that is noninvasive, non-manipulative, and really might bring comfort in ways that they couldn't.

What I bring to oncology, or have brought to oncology, was the sense of connecting to people, no matter what their story is, no matter how rough they may be on the outside; the gift is seeing their highest self and potential and always reaching for that and knowing it's a privilege to do that. And obviously, there were patients that had been difficult, you know, and really challenged me more, but I did not give up on them or on that belief that there's still a higher self to connect with that deserves dignity and respect.

So, you know, before you knew it, I received many awards for my work and psychosocial programs. If I presented at an Oncology conference, I wrote a small article for our Cancer Center newsletter with pictures of me to keep my teams informed. It also became a reminder to refer patients stating: "Hey, go see Marsha!" In addition what we started in our Rad/Onc social work group was a short intake form, because despite 1:1 referrals we were missing people; we didn't want to leave referrals just to our doctors and nurses who were so busy, or maybe had their own blind spots about issues. We had the patients self-refer by answering the following: Did you need counseling? Did you need family intervention? Did you need stress reduction? Did you want Reiki? I started putting the word down Reiki instead of just stress reduction; it helped us to educate and better explain what a Reiki session might be like. Did you have issues with death and dying? Did you need resources? So, it just became more and more acceptable seeing a social worker.

When Susan G. Coleman Race for the Cure offered grants for programs, I was very naive and thought one could just ask for funds to be used as needed; not so and there was a whole grant application process. My first program was music for recovery and congruence with breast cancer; the music therapist I was going to work with said I had to be part of the pro-

gram, and I had to help. I had to write the grant with her. It was pretty remarkable. Some of my support group women participated as well as others. We also did retreats. Drumming from these programs helped to create our protocol when children finished radiation to walk in the Cancer Center with drums and bubbles. Since I was the 1st social worker in the country who, I believe, was also a Reiki master teacher, I later put in a grant to teach minority and non-minority women with breast cancer Reiki level one for stress reduction and healing. When I knew I was going to put in for a grant, I honestly remember myself pacing back and forth questioning and reflecting upon what would get funded, and all these different ideas kept coming through. And the right one came through, and I got the grant. Part of the program was doing a retreat up at Whispering Hope Ranch in Payson. It was incredibly cool to be able to do this as a social worker. At the ranch we worked on animals that had special needs; they were animals that were there to help special need populations. I wrote about this experience and then presented on it at an Oncology conference and also at a poster session. And then after the grant concluded, my manager allowed me to teach some follow-up classes so that more cancer survivors, not just breast cancer survivors, could learn Reiki.

Wisdom to Share to Clinicians Going into Oncology

It's like you can't just stay under the radar. You also have to plant seeds all the time and not be afraid to tell your story. Tell your narrative. Stand out with what you know is your expertise. Don't be scared to have an expertise. That's because we all can do something unique that will create value and joy. Be the person your staff and patients and families can come to.

I was really fortunate that when I started at the Cancer Center they agreed to send me to one conference a year. I highly recommend this to stay fresh, form connections, and increase one's skills. If you learn one new tool, it has been valuable and may also replenish you. Upon coming back don't be afraid, as I said, to find your voice and share things with your team. For example, at our weekly interdisciplinary meetings, I almost always, unless they were running late, would say "excuse me" at the end: "I'd like to just share something." Perhaps I would share about a new resource or a group opportunity. Or following attending a conference on psychosexuality, I would begin a brief conversation about how to address this issue with patients. Some of our doctors came up to me later stating: "If we need to do it, we'll call you instead to do this." I didn't care, because not everyone has the same comfort level or training; what is most important however is that they know whom to go to and not block this out. It's a topic and issue that's important in people's lives.

What Does Your Specific Profession Bring to Patients?

As an undergraduate student I learned the importance and power of words after being a hypnosis subject at the Brooklyn VA. How one uses words and reframes words can make huge differences in coping.

It started me on doing more visualization with clients to help them to better cope with their treatments, stressors, and to find inner peace. Teaching breathwork is also a skill that social workers can teach to our clients and staff. And again, we can teach individuals to be more mindful. What is mindfulness? It's helping to get people off of the narrative and the negative meaning they attach to pain or fear, or their projections into the future. We can then help get them back into breath and being present in the here and now with compassion.

Can we come up with or co-create an imagery that could be more peaceful and feel safer? That's part of what led me along and helped me to support so many clients facing oncology challenges.

Some people have very large families, and I didn't go to everyone's funeral. My recommendation is unless it's part of your job, you're not going to want to. You can't be all things to all people at all times.

But I remember one of my Oncology docs called me at home; a community VIP's wife had just died; he was from a very large family, and they were not doing well. He asked me to go out to their home. And I'm thinking, "Oh, my goodness, I don't know these people, and I am walking into one of the darkest periods of their lives." I think our profession teaches us to walk into almost anything, and to try to have grace and skill. This is the same skill set to listen, identify needs, and provide support. I had to sense out what are these individuals needing? What are they feeling? Sometimes it's verbal. Sometimes it's not. Sometimes it's getting people to talk to each other. Sometimes it's reading a poem; so much depends upon ages, culture, and circumstances. We have such a variety of skills available. I remember with this family, and this would not have been who I am with my upbringing, but I knew they were very religious. There were 22 people, and I asked them to hold hands together with me, and we started out by praying. It was what was needed, and then I facilitated that session to work as a support group engaged in sharing grief, loss, and healing memories. You're meeting individuals where they are at and where they need to be at that moment. Social work, I think, is an amazing.

I'm still always learning. My clients were always teaching me, and I always tried not to be stale; if you find yourself dreading your work for more than brief periods, get out of the field.

Go into working at a boutique store or something. There's many ways we could live a life of value. We want to be fresh. Our clients deserve it, and just the variety of skills we have can provide us with many social work opportunities. We can meet the needs of our clients in different ways, and that's different for each client. I talk about having your own treasure chest, because what's good for one person is definitely not for another. I remember going in to see someone in the hospital whom one of the docs from ICU asked me to see. He had cancer and had a lot of pain. I anticipated that I would offer him perhaps breathwork or Reiki. The doc had asked me to do Reiki on him, and he just looked at me and said, "I'm not interested." I chose to stay a few minutes, being respectful and assessing if there might be a shift and if there was something he was willing to accept from my Social Work visit. I said, "Is there anything I can do for you today?" And he said, "no." I said, "Thank you for sharing your time." I left with something my former Reiki master teacher taught me—to not get attached to an outcome. And that's sometimes hard, because we care about our clients and want to make a difference; we think we'd like it to look a certain way or support dying to be perhaps a little easier, or for a family issue to be resolved. You know we can only do the best we can in a circumstance, and that's pretty darn good. That is truly good and meaningful.

In terms of most memorable experiences, "And I was thinking about that. And the comparison was that if I go to an Indian restaurant I prefer the buffet. Don't give me one dish. I like to taste things and enjoy the variety of tastes and flavors. So, I'm not going to come up with a favorite because each stage of my career, each opportunity was such a gift in retrospect. It was perhaps like the news media coming in which scared the heck out of me, but it also gave me a chance to really prepare to do this, learn a new skill, and grow.

I got the Ben's Bell for kindness. That was my best award. I got other awards. But to be acknowledged by your patients and staff for being kind, even though this is just who we are; it felt amazing to be seen and recognized for, knowing that not everyone works in a profession where staying present and being kind are such prerequisites.

So, as I was preparing to finish up working in Oncology at the hospital after being there for thirty-six-and-a-half years, I reflected on the people I had met and touched and programs I had created. Looking at it all, it truly felt like it was a great "gig." And I say this with all respect, because I felt so much gratitude and pride. I achieved a lot. I had the opportunity to change some of the climate of the hospital. I taught doctors, nurses, and therapists as well as MSW interns and colleagues about psychosocial issues and needs as well as about psychosexuality; that was pretty wonderful. And, I knew it felt complete; I felt really good. That whisper from within, however, said, "You are going to dance your way out from this place on your last day."

I thought my husband, who loved tango at that time was going to come to clinic, and we were going to dance out of radiation oncology to tango. Well, he didn't come. So much for that vision. Okay, but my daughter Rachael came. One of our oncologists had given all of us in Rad/Onc (Radiation Oncology) small bottles of champagne for Christmas; I had saved mine. I sat out in the Diamond Children's garden outside, and I had already given in my badge.

It was like they took away my privileges. I'm finished, they basically said, you're done, you know. So … I sat outside sipping a little champagne and just acknowledging and reflecting upon this momentous day. It's important to take time to reflect on our lives and accomplishments. We need to feel grateful. We need to acknowledge, even on the bad days, what went well and what I was able to do. That you know is something we don't do enough of. I believe that we can really be hard on ourselves as social workers; it's time to change that.

And then in that garden I remembered that I was definitely going to dance out of the hospital to say "goodbye." However, there was a problem; I was already outside. I just knew something didn't feel complete. And then all of a sudden, I looked down. My pocketbook which I had put down to take photos was missing. I thought that someone had stolen it, so I had to go back in the hospital to security to find out and request assistance. This turn of events was a blessing because I had really wanted to thank security for all their help over the years with my groups and retreats. So I go inside and thank goodness, of course my bag was there; a bit of an orchestration from the universe.

I express my gratitude, and I'm thinking, "Okay, I still need to dance out even if it feels a bit sacrilegious." I put on my phone the song Celebrate. And I start to dance out through the lobby with people surprised and hopefully somewhat amused. Perhaps some thought I was a bit crazy; it didn't matter. What was important was that it was important to celebrate oneself. And I danced out on the balcony of the hospital, and it was my goodbye to this incredible journey and a step forward onto the next chapter of my life journey. This one now was fully complete.

I highly recommend that we each find a way (you don't have to dance.) You may think that Marsha could do it because she's bold and a little crazy. I actually was pretty shy, and was not initially comfortable doing these things. It's about allowing oneself to keep developing and growing. Let the lessons from one's patients on being authentic come out and guide you on your own unique and precious way.

CHAPTER 5

Ana Maria Lopez, MD, MPH

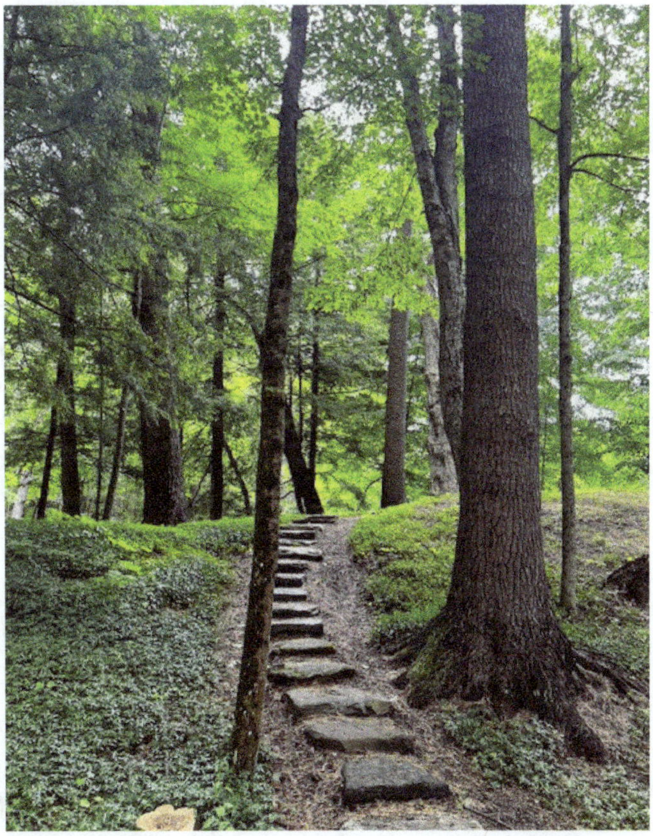

Dr. Lopez's persona reflects her patience, kindness, and her being present. She leads with empathy and understanding and has a gift of listening. I was fortunate to have met her as an MSW intern at the Arizona Cancer Center. She always referred her patients to social work with a deep understanding of the importance of psychosocial care. She always listened to her patients and was able to give me great information from what she learned. I was always impressed by her ability to show her expertise and brilliance in the field of medical oncology. In turn, she always shared with me the medical side of what our patients were facing.

I was extremely fortunate to have had one of the greatest opportunities to be a senior research specialist for Dr. Lopez. She was passionate about addressing all aspects of her patients' overall well-being as she was studying various aspects of psychosocial care. I was able to learn about the importance of research and passion. I was able to work with her on a mindfulness-based stress reduction study for women with stage II breast cancer. I also supported a study comparing the impact of self-directed exercise on women going through breast cancer treatment. One group walked on their own, and the other group did NIA (Neuromuscular Interactive Action) together. We found in comparing their blood analysis and self-reports that there are more benefits to the self-directed exercise (NIA). This was my first opportunity to know the significance of research and how I could be involved to impact the field of social work and oncology healthcare.

Dr. Lopez always supported my learning and passions. She was influential in writing my first book on the interviews of my patients and their families who went through pediatric bone marrow transplant. She was my support and mentor. I increased my knowledge of research and my writing skills.

Throughout my career, I have published articles on cancer, grief and loss, and posttraumatic growth. I know my passion for being a part of research is because of my work with Dr. Lopez. I feel grateful for her guidance and challenging me to be a clinician plus participate in research.

In April of 2024, Dr. Lopez and I reconnected at University of Arizona's Integrative Health Summit (Dr. Weil's). Not only did I get to visit with her, but I personally met Dr. Kabat-Zinn, the founder of Mindfulness-Based Stress Reduction. She and I spoke and connected on our careers, and this conversation inspired the thoughts that led to the writing of this book. Not only that, I am also now participating in her research providing MBSR training for her breast cancer patients.

During this interview, I felt honored to see her confidence and assurance that the impact she is making is deeply routed in providing comprehensive care to her patients. She values inspiring her residents and colleagues by demonstrating the incorporation of programs and research.

Being able to have the time to ask her these questions was very powerful as I listened. To be able to be present to see her development from a new oncologist to now one with wisdom and patience and a focus of being present was perceptive.

Why Did You Go into Oncology?

> *I'm a medical oncologist, and I initially decided on cancer care. When I was a resident, I had at some point decided that it was going to be adult medicine and not pediatrics because I just thought pediatrics would be too hard. Pediatricians are saints.*
>
> *And I was thinking between oncology and cardiology. And I remember talking with some of my mentors and trying to figure that out. And then what I realized is that I really liked the intensity of emotional connection and intellectual stimulation that oncology has, at least for me, and that was really important. I was a philosophy major as an undergraduate. And one of the big things that I would study or think about is, you know, how humans are aware that they're going to die. And how incredibly intense it is when a person realizes*

this. I think we all know we're going to die, but often, when there's a diagnosis of cancer, there's the proximity of death that people need to face. How I felt is what a privilege to be able to walk with people during that time, and to be able to help them in any way possible. And, their families, as they go through that. So, that emotional connection and at the same time, you know, you're trying to help them with the stressors facing their physical body, their emotional health, and whatever other issues they're having. So being able to address the whole person.

I loved the fact that Dr. Lopez knew from an early age she wanted to be a doctor and help people. And for her to really fulfill her dream.

For a long time, I remember being in elementary school, and somebody would fall in the playground, and I would go and try to take care of where they got hurt. So, in that sense, I think I really wanted to take care of people from a very early age.

Dr. Lopez recalls part of an interview that she chose to talk about an influential oncology patient out of all the patients she had seen. The interviewer noticed how she was interested in oncology at the point. I also find it fascinating that her role as a medical oncologist is focused on that connection with patients during a really hard time and not just the intelligence of treating the cancer.

What Is Your Personal Meaning from Oncology?

I think that on the one hand, the cancer diagnosis is very scary for people. On the other hand, there's been tremendous progress (medical treatment). Although that progress is in the statistics, the outcome for that individual patient is still individual.

I mean, there are situations where a 5% survival rate is "expected," but for the patient it might be 100% because they may be in that 5%. And I think about how to keep people connected with that sense of possibility regardless of where they are. And, despite all the progress, there are still those situations that we don't fully understand. There are people with metastatic disease who are living for years and years and years. Even though I believe the statistics, I am very much supportive of my patient, and where they are. That is to say, you know, from where we are right now, these are all possible paths for you. I don't know which one's going to be the one, but I'm going to be with you the whole way. And, then, to be there. Another thing that I have thought about around this experience is the concept of compassion. Thinking about the root of the word, to be with in their suffering. The being with is healing for both of us. It is something.

From our conversation I remembered that she taught me this as an intern. And it just really helped me find hope in the work I do. I never knew what percentage my patients were in and that gave me a sense of promise in all situations. After working with Dr. Lopez, I went into pediatric BMT, and many of the kids I attended to had cancer for years, and they were in despair, and I went to work keeping that perspective that there is hope. Just within the past month, I purchased a wedding gift for my very first pediatric oncology patient. That is so beautiful.

> *People say to me, "Aren't you burned out?" or "How do you protect yourself?" I don't feel like I need to protect myself. Honestly, I just really feel like the being there with that person; that's just a tremendous privilege, to be able to be there, and to walk with them. It's not anything extraordinary. I'm just walking with, but it's incredible and sustaining for both of us.*

Dr. Lopez really exemplifies true meaning in her work. To be able to be present with patients as they face death is very meaningful, and it takes a special person to feel that honor with each interaction.

What Insight Did You Gain from Your Work?

> *I think that everybody's path is really unique, and at the same time, it's really human. I'm a breast oncologist. So probably 99% of the people I've cared for have been women. I've been doing more integrative oncology in the last few years, and I'm seeing men. There are so many similarities. We're all human. People want to be supported. I feel like people are people; people are human, and we all seek understanding and comfort. I think a lot about being with the patient where they are. That often means checking in with them to see what would bring greatest comfort. I often say, "We could try this if you'd like, or I could sit with you as you go through this, if you would like." It's just checking in with them. "You tell me what would work for you."*
>
> *It's not a prescriptive thing. I will be with you in the way that works for you. So sometimes people may, you know, for whatever reasons they may be a little reticent. And that's okay. Then, it's just my job to let them know that "I 'm here for you." Ultimately, it's their life. It's their choice and how they want to proceed with it. It's a universal human experience, but how people go through it is really individual. And, how to respect that is important.*
>
> *Currently, in healthcare, there's a push to formalize and standardize. There's an effort to standardize patient communication.*

For example, if somebody dies, there's a standard note to send. I wonder if that takes away the heart, the human connection that was built when caring for the individual and their family.

You know, they (the communication) would just have to be different, because it's tailored to that person.

What I share with the students, the residents, and the fellows is that it's an experience of tremendous gratitude to be able to be there with a patient.

Dr. Lopez always had the insight of knowing that you just really have to empower the patients. Give them your options and medical advice, but then listen to their fears and concerns—to be able to really hear what they are experiencing. That is a gift and mindset that Dr. Lopez creates.

Memorable Moments to Share

There's been, I think, a lot of change since I was a fellow. In general, the research focus for the fellow in medical oncology is and has been on drug development. My focus was on quality of life and cancer prevention and community partnership, so I didn't quite fit the mold.

I remember the very 1st grant that I wrote, and it was on quality of life. I sent in the protocol, and it came back, totally red. It was completely marked up. That was in the days of paper submissions. Unknowingly, I went to meet with the review people to be sure that I understood the comments, and, I guess, nobody had ever done that. I remember feeling really awful after that experience, because the message that I took away was—this work was going nowhere. I really needed to think about drug development.

At the time, I was in Tucson, and it must have been wintertime because when I had gotten there it was dark, and I was taking the stairs in the cancer center where there are windows. I remember walking back after that meeting, I was just feeling very down and feeling like my career was going nowhere, and as I'm walking up the stairs—it was just a spiritual moment. As I'm going up the stairs, and I'm starting to see light of the day through the windows, and I realized, wait, I'm doing this study, because this is what I'm hearing from patients. Patients were saying, "Why do we want this treatment if we're going to feel so awful? If we don't have quality of life, we don't want it."

And I realize. That's right. If you don't have quality of life, what do you have? It was a great moment. I'm walking up the stairs. The sun is coming up. And I'm feeling stronger and stronger as I'm walking up the stairs and thinking, "This is right. This is science."

I feel that I've learned so much from my patients through the experience of connecting with them, listening to them, and asking, from their lens, "How could this be better?"

I've been able to share these lessons with my mentees. I recently spoke with a young woman who is maybe a few years out of fellowship, and she was talking about how she wanted to focus on a patient education intervention and in speaking with others, she had been discouraged from this work because it wasn't funded. So, she walked away resigned to not pursuing her work. We spoke, and I encouraged her not to give up on a good idea, and to think about what could be done even without funding. She walked away saying, "Oh, wow! I guess that's true. I can do this."

Dr. Lopez is persistent and never gives up. She is an advocate for her patients in creating research and programs that enhance their quality of life. In a medical setting where there is pressure to spend less time with patients and, instead, to work toward drug development, she instills her value of listening to her patients. She never gives up on developing programs and support for them.

Like this weekend, it was a small thing, but it made a difference. I happened to speak with a community member at an event, and she was wanting to put together a health fair. We spoke about logistics, connected her to the right folks, and then engaged medical students who really helped make it happen. I really do love listening to what people would like and then coming up ways to just make it happen.

I think that's part of where I am right now. I really feel that it's important to support others' and their dreams. I mean, I'm not going to work much longer, probably. I always say—"life is short, and the work is long." So, the only way that we can really make an impact is to support the next generation. I feel really, really committed to that. I hope that I'm planting seeds that will hopefully give birth to trees whose shade I'll never sit under. But that's the goal, right? The intent is that those seeds that are planted grow and blossom and go on to make more seeds. It's the only way that we can continue the change.

This is so beautiful—the imagery and belief in hope and impact. I really think Dr. Lopez's essence of mindfulness stems from her values.

What Do You Do for Self-care?

> *I think I do not often feel burned out or stressed because of my connection and presence with the patient, with the mentee, with my life. For me, the experience is spiritual, transcendental. It's almost like I tap into something deeper that is an inexhaustible energy.*

Dr. Lopez finds meaning in the spiritual connection to her patients. This allows for her to be energized by these moments.

> *I'm not often thinking, "Oh, work is so stressful. I need to do something else." But, I do think about self-care. What's been different for me in the last several years is to think about being present. There was a time when I prized the fact that I could multitask. I would envision myself being and doing multiple roles all happening at the same time. Now, I think about being present with a person, with the book I'm reading, or even when I'm watching TV. I seek to be present with whatever I'm doing. That by itself makes for a different experience. I don't think the word is relaxing. I think it's actually energizing. For example, when I walk, I'm rarely listening to a podcast. I focus on being on my walk. I appreciate the air and the birds, and, whatever comes my way. Similarly, if I'm eating, I try to take those few minutes to be present with my eating. And I really feel that this has helped me not to stress.*

This is the essence of mindfulness.

Wisdom to Share to Clinicians Going into Oncology

> *I am working on a curriculum for students on well-being. I realize that it's the same as what I emphasize with patients.*
>
> *"Eat well," I tell them, "eat well, sleep well, and find joy." You know, that's the key.*
>
> *There are so many stressors for young people, and so how to help them to be present, not to panic and to take care of themselves. And to just start. Now.*
>
> *I really do think that it's the one-on-one. The one-on-one with the patient. The one-on-one with the student, the mentee, the other person.*
>
> *I would love to see a kind and gentle healthcare system. That's not what exists. Hopefully, through the one-on-one and by role-modeling, patients, students, and trainees can see*

another path. Changing hearts and minds is a one-on-one effort, and at the same time, working in the advocacy space and working within the health system. But ultimately, the one-on-one changes hearts and minds.

Dr. Lopez believes that one connection can make an impact of a more accessible and human focused care. I love that she is hopeful and gives concrete ways to accomplish this. Teaching students and fellows to practice mindfulness in their work. Not only does that impact patients, it can transcend to medical care system.

How Do You Rationalize Cancer?

It's absolutely not fair, absolutely not.

But there is likely a human-made component in what has been done to the environment, to the food system, to how we live. I encourage people to think about the basics. Eat food that you have cooked. Eat food that your grandmother would recognize as food. There are lots of things that we can eat because we're omnivores. but that doesn't mean it's food. And, be active and limit your stress. I mean, people are really stressed, so we need to help people to limit their stress. Find joy. Laugh!

I read somewhere that you only need 10%, to spend 10% of your time in something that nurtures you. That's not a lot. Encouraging people to find joy, meaning at the starting dose of 10% of your time. Maybe it's a 10-minute walk. If you're really present, it can feel like a vacation. By being present and enjoying what comes your way—seeing little kids, a puppy can bring a smile. Allow that part of your soul to be happy by finding joy in the moment. All of this can help reverse the inflammation, some of the toxicity.

So, cancer risk from the environment and lifestyle is human-made. In that same way, it could be human-unmade by how we live as individuals and by advocating for change. We have to put our energy towards that.

What Is the Most Impactful Part of Your Career?

As a physician, we have these built-in divisions. You're the medical oncologist. You're the radiation oncologist. You're the dermatologist. You're the endocrinologist, and so on. The goal, it seems, is for everyone to stay in their own lane. This often means that nobody is taking care of the whole person. As the medical oncologist, you often become the patient's primary doc. That may mean connecting the dots with the other docs or with the pharmacy or the insurance. It may not be glamorous, and it's not reimbursed, but it's an important role, essential for the person's care.

For example, a call, a simple check-in can help care so much. "Just wanted to be sure you picked up your meds." "Have you started the new medicine? Is it going okay?"

By thinking of the patient as a whole person, I see part of my job as helping the patient get care. Getting care is not easy.

I appreciate the vision of change one patient at a time. And having this perspective can make systematic change in how we support patients with cancer.

Anything Else You Want to Share?

I think I feel better after this conversation! Thank you for that.

I might get choked up. At my core, I feel what a tremendous privilege and honor it is to be a doctor. Just be able to be there with people and to help them in their time of need is just an honor.

There have been changes that I've seen during my career that have made it harder for people to get care. On the other hand, as I reflect on it, it hasn't impeded care. By being there for people, by taking care of your patients the way you'd want your mother to be taken care, that's the goal. And if you do that, people feel it. It is a tremendous honor to care for patients. You helped me to reconnect with that feeling.

CHAPTER 6

Carolann Dougherty Mashouf

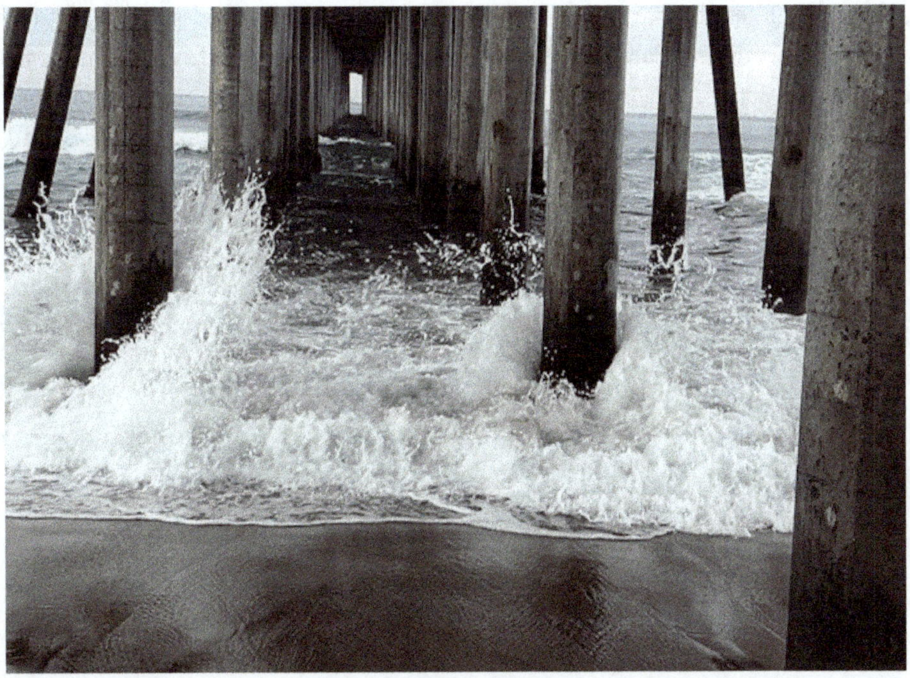

Carolann has the gift of spreading and welcoming happiness. When I first met her at the Arizona Cancer Center, I was still an MSW intern. Just being around her made me feel heard and present. Carolann still has this ability. She is so positive and happy. When I was discovering my role in my internship, everyday she would smile and thank me for being there. Carolann always made me feel welcome and introduced me to her patients. She validated the need for social work for her patients. That feeling she always shared with others made me realize she is a chemo angel. I used to tell my patients the chemo nurses are angels, and I know she truly is.

Why Did You Go into Oncology?

Carolann stared her nursing career on an IV team in the late 1970s, and they happened, at that time, to give chemo. She thinks back to how they did this without any precautions, gloves, masks, and so on! But there was some really strong connection with patients she had been giving the chemo. Carolann naturally always had a good stick, but sitting down and talking to her patients, that was where the meaning was for her.

> *I love the essence of sitting down and talking to patients. While you're giving them treatment, you know I really loved that. It was amazing to me.*

In her job, she really likes the part of giving chemo because she could sit and talk to her patients while giving the medications. Carolann even ran a support group, without training, while working in a small oncology practice. She learned so much but wished she had more skills to run the group. Being there and listening to the patients is where she really gained her experience. And she continued that support, listening to patients while giving chemo, throughout her career. She alludes to the fact that it was just part of her personality, getting to know her cancer patients.

> *It's a very powerful thing when you can sit down and really have deep conversations. Not just about cancer disease and treatment. Let's take it deeper; patients need so much more than simply discussing their disease and treatment.*

Carolann had that intrinsic need to be there for her patients and really connect. She got nationally certified in oncology nursing soon after realizing her passion.

What Is Your Personal Meaning from Oncology?

Carolann shares how doing this work impacted her whole life.

> *It brought my life into a much deeper perspective. My career made my life so much fuller. It made me appreciate every day. You know ... just any little problem you have. It's like nothing compared to what you see.*

Carolann shared how working with other passionate oncology nurses and doctors really made her feel appreciative and appreciated. Something about the dedication and appreciation of the work we do and how it connects us together. Her happiness in how she worked always shone through.

> *My colleagues understood the essence of life. They appreciate every day.*

Carolann shares why the work is so real.

> *I think that cancer patients are staring their mortality right in the face. They know that every day you have to make each day count.*

This insight about the meaning, and knowing how life and health are precious, reflects a deep connection that oncology healthcare providers share. Seeing what we see, we intrinsically know this and live it. Learning from what our patients go through, I believe this is part of the dedication oncology professionals possess and carry it into their personal lives.

What Insights Did You Gain from Your Work?

Carolann shares her view that when patients experience pain, her focus or that of clinicians is not so much about their pain; instead, it is the effect that pain has on their quality of life and how it brings them to a deeper meaning in all that they do. And from her work, Carolann knows it is important to "smell the roses." We don't have forever, and our time on earth is precious. This insight impacts the way in which she lives and appreciates her life.

How Do You Handle the Loss, Sadness, and Grief?

In respect to this, Carolann understands the balance of life.

> *I have to embrace every day and have other interests outside of work, because balance in life was so necessary. That was important in my career to help keep me healthy mentally and physically.*

So, for Carolann, having this foundation of understanding through the sadness helped. She also took action into supporting her nursing colleagues by creating a sympathy card program. When someone died, a card was sent to their family, which helped with closure and support to both her colleagues and the patient's loved ones. Even thought this wasn't part of her job criteria, she developed this so that nurses could have an outlet when losing patients. Not only did she spearhead this at work; she got her community involved as well. Carolann got donations from a Hallmark store for the cards. This brings awareness of what cancer patients and their families go through. It establishes a community. These were secondary impacts she created, but what follows was her main objective:

It was my intent for the patient's family to know we, the cancer center staff, remembered and acknowledged the loss of their loved one.

Carolann would send a card on behalf of the Cancer Center staff in hopes the family would know that they cared.

Carolann also was an avid walker, and got outdoors every day. Something about being outdoors, in nature, gave her that balance.

Walking just cleared my head and it brought such peace to my soul which turned me into an avid walker.

Memorable Moments to Share?

Carolann took initiative and started a bubble program for patients. When they finished their last chemo treatment, they would have a bubble ceremony in the chemo room to celebrate the event. All of the nurses and available staff surrounded the patient and would blow bubbles. It's a memorable event to the patient, their family, and the staff.

She also created an aftercare packet for patients. She contacted Dr. Andrew Weil's Integrative Medicine clinic and collaborated to give patients more support and resources. Carolann's actions made an impact of change and community support. She took initiative to make positive program changes for her colleagues and patients.

Her most impactful influence was implementing a cancer specialty boutique at the Arizona Cancer Center in Tucson, Arizona. Carolann wanted to have a place where a woman could go and get breast prosthesis, wig, and other supportive needs right where they were being treated. This vision took a long time and effort after many said no to her vision. But Carolann never gave up. And this boutique continues to provide support for cancer patients.

Carolann was also perceptive to the support the center provided for caregivers. She knew caregivers needed additional support and were not receiving it. So, she created a resource pack for them to get the information they needed.

In her career, Carolann would see a need and then develop a solution to implement it. This has, and continues to have, a profound impact for patients and colleagues to this day.

Not only did she create this boutique; she even helped with the development of a fashion show for patients and their families. Her oncology nursing association and community stores would donate time and clothes. It was a celebration of the patients and a good community event that brought happiness to many patients and their families.

> *It was called "Embrace Change." The patients LOVED it as did their families. It was so fun and therapeutic for all of us to have this wonderful experience.*

In our discussion, Carolann looks back at the experiences of her patients.

> *It's all a very personal experience. One of the things that I always admired was my patients who had great faith. When they faced adversity, the bad news, they would turn to God. Their faith helped them deal with disappointment and anger which helped them cope. Of course, we had patients that had a very hard time dealing with their diagnosis and treatment. But across the board, faith-based patients and their families coped better. I always admired them greatly and thought I've got to personally work on my faith.*

Carolann and I discussed a mutual patient and her impact. She was young, newly married, vibrant, and beautiful. But her essence after the diagnosis turned to pure fear. She was so needy and scared. Losing her made us as a staff so sad, and we continue to carry her memory with us to this day.

What Do You Do for Self-care?

Carolann was fortunate to work part-time, and she feels that gave her more of a balanced life. It allowed space for the hard work as well as time for self-care and her family. But, as we know, not everyone in oncology has that opportunity.

She would attend events created by the pharmaceutical companies as well as educational oncology conferences. This was helpful for her to have some time with her colleagues outside of work.

Personally, attending a funeral was very hard for her, so she was selective and cautious about that.

Carolann has a deep connection with God, and personal beliefs were helpful to her self-care.

Meaning of Mindfulness in Oncology Care

Carolann has that ability to be present with her patients. But it wasn't always the case. Early in her career, she didn't know what to say. And she says, "You never know what will trigger people." But leading with listening and kindness is always the way. She was meeting with a patient who was very sick from the chemo and she was trying to offer encouragement.

"It's nice that you're older and have lived your life." Carolann realized that was the wrong thing to say!! The patient responded, *"What do you mean? I know I'm older, but I deserve to live."* That's a lesson one never forgets.

What Have You Personally Brought to Oncology Care?

"Truly, I felt that I was a voice for the patients and their advocate."

Not only was she an amazing good stick and provided support during chemotherapy treatments, Carolann made program changes to support her patients and their families.

Wisdom to Share to Clinicians Going into Oncology

Carolann advises clinicians to *"just show up and be present."* Being there for patients and meeting them where they are and listening to their stories and the meaning behind them.

> *When you don't know what to say, when you really don't know what to say, simply say, "I really have no words. I don't know what to say, because this is so difficult and sad." Be honest and be there. Listen to what they say and respond accordingly.*

I would tell clinicians that *"it's more of a calling. It's not a job."*

And to always remember:

> *My career was life-changing to me, showing me the importance of appreciating every day that we live. As my career went on, I realized more and more the importance of self-care. We as nurses are horrible at that. We are good at caring for others, but not for ourselves.*

What Does Your Profession Bring to Oncology Care?

Caring for oncology patients is very intimate. The trust that develops in these relationships is very intense. I was always a very cautious nurse. I think it's my training over the many years. I really loved orienting and teaching new nurses. That was amazing and challenging to me. And I couldn't stress the importance enough to my colleagues about administering chemotherapy drugs. You can give them a hundred times to a patient and can still have a serious drug reaction. You always need to be prepared for that.

How Does She Rationalize Cancer?

"I couldn't do the work I did if I didn't know there was a heaven."

What Has Been the Most impactful Part of Your Career?

My goodbyes at the cancer center, it was so hard to walk away. It was gut-wrenching. I knew it was time for me to enjoy my grandchildren, downsize my life, and time to move on to life's next chapter. But still, it was so hard to walk away. I walked out of the cancer center crying, especially saying goodbye to my patients, colleagues, and the boutique.

CHAPTER 7

Erika Meneely, CNP

This interview was just meant to be. I have always believed that people are placed in your life for a reason. I have never worked with Erika directly, but I was the social worker at Massachusetts General Hospital on the same team, colorectal. I connected with Erika from a long-term family friend who was going through cancer treatment. She was enthusiastic about how incredible Erika was; so, I reached out. I was unsure, since it would be the first person I interviewed who I didn't work with in my career.

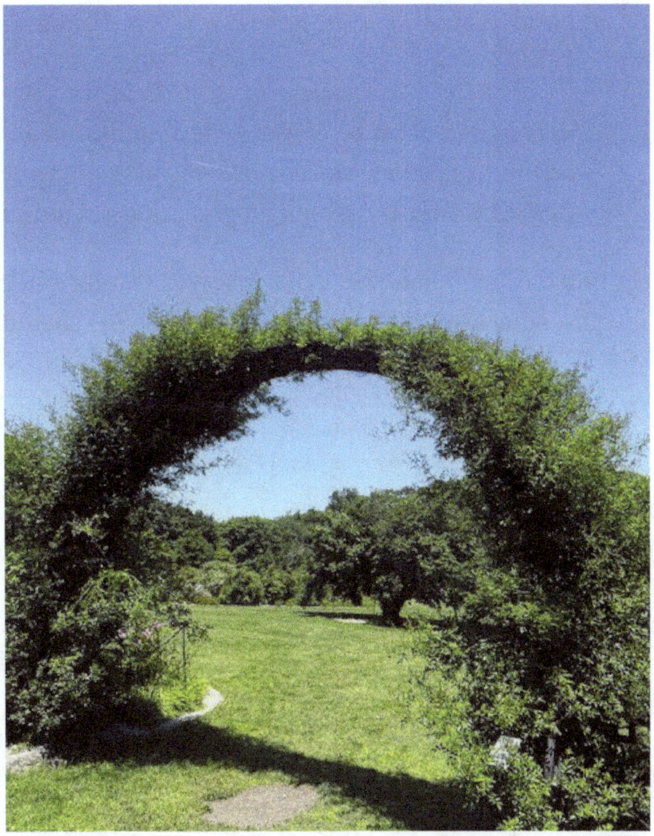

But this interaction was meaningful and really beautiful, and I feel the lessons that Erika shared really elevated this book's insight. She is honest and real and has a deep dedication to her patients. She is present and real with them.

It was a definite honor that she took the time to share her incredible career, and to be able to listen to her experience was inspiring.

Why Did You Go into Oncology?

When Erika first graduated from college she worked for public television. She communicated with many high-profile people, including Hodding Carter, Assistant Secretary of State for Public Affairs by President Jimmy Carter, and Bill Moyers. This was an exciting first post-graduation job for a young person.

> *I had a challenging time choosing a field of study and explored several majors at St. Anselm College. Throughout my college years, I frequently expressed a desire to become a nurse. However, my father's response was, "You don't want to be a nurse. You don't want to empty bedpans." Taking his advice into account, I graduated with a degree in criminal justice. This led me to a career in public television, where I worked on the documentary series FRONTLINE.*
>
> *It didn't feel like the right fit, so I decided to pursue my long-standing wish to return to nursing school. At 24, it was quite an adjustment. I left a stable job and a steady income to become a full-time student. Having already earned my bachelor's degree from St. Anselm College, I chose a diploma program that I could complete in two years.*

I think it is honorable that Erika followed her gut and pursued a career she really wanted. This is the beginning of a very meaningful profession. She shared she has been in nursing for over 30 years.

What Is Your Personal Meaning from Oncology?

> *I realized early on that I wanted a career in oncology. When I was 10 years old, my mother was diagnosed with breast cancer. Over the course of six years, she endured numerous surgeries and treatments. She was only thirty-five when she passed away, and I was sixteen.*

It was an incredibly challenging time. Losing my mom at 16 was profoundly difficult, as people often recognize. Yet, as an adult, I find it even harder not having her here. Reaching significant milestones in my life, I deeply wish she were here to share those moments with me.

Reflecting back, I remember the doctors were frequently in and out of the hospital while my mother was sick. They provided expert care and did everything they could, but it was the nurses who were truly present. They were at the bedside with us every day, deeply engaged with our family. They understood our family dynamics, offered comfort, and absorbed our pain. Alongside the advances in science, medicine, and technology, it was the nurses' compassion and support that stood out. This experience solidified my decision to pursue a career in oncology. It's what I've always wanted to do.

I want to be a resource for others in the way I felt supported during my own experience.

With such a profound loss it is so touching how she was called to be an oncology nurse. And to just be able to have gone through it, she intrinsically understands what pains, emotional and physical, cancer patients and their families go through. It's an unfortunate gift but also a blessing to be able to have that connection.

What Insight Did You Gain from Your Work?

A cancer diagnosis is frightening and affects not just the patient but also their family members. I deeply empathize with what my patients and their families are going through. Over the years, I initially thought it unprofessional to show emotion in front of patients. However, I realized that my emotions stem from genuine care. Caring for someone often means forming a relationship that can last for years. It's natural to feel sadness when someone you've grown close to is suffering, in pain, or nearing the end of their life. I no longer feel embarrassed about this. As I've gained more experience in my career, I've become more comfortable expressing to my patients that I care about them, and that's because I truly do.

In my role as a nurse practitioner, I not only provide medical recommendations but also focus on building meaningful relationships with my patients. Despite their own emotional and physical suffering, they often ask about me and my family. They genuinely share in my joys and celebrate the good moments with me.

Given that much of their time is consumed by clinic visits, managing the side effects of cancer treatment, and discussing their illness, patients greatly welcome the opportunity to talk about topics beyond cancer. We work together through challenging conversations about goals of care and end-of-life issues. It is a profound privilege to share this intimate space with them, even though it is difficult to face the impending loss. I am deeply touched when patients express concern for my well-being and recognize the emotional weight of delivering difficult news. I see my role as guiding patients through this transition from life to the next, and I strive to make that journey as uncomplicated as possible.

I strive to make the journey easier for patients. Some may argue that I don't always set strict boundaries, but I see my weekend and evening phone calls as a form of volunteering. While some people contribute by working at a soup kitchen or donating to causes, I believe that being available to answer calls and provide support outside of regular hours offer patients reassurance and a sense of safety. For me, this is a meaningful way to give back.

Erika has definitely made this work a gratitude of giving and, in turn, she gets back from her patients their gratitude for her. It is evident she makes the work align with her needs and sets her own boundaries in her job that feel right for her.

Memorable Moments to Share

This really resonates that Erika is able to be with people where they are at and allow for their choices.

> *Throughout my 30-year career, I've experienced countless memorable moments and met many remarkable people. Some individuals have touched my life more profoundly than others, and I will always carry their memory with me. I think of them on their birthdays, the anniversaries of their passing, or whenever I encounter a gift that reminds me of them.*
>
> *One indelible memory from my early nursing career involves a patient named Mattie, who had leukemia and was frequently hospitalized for extended periods. Despite her frail appearance, she had an incredible strength and a remarkably positive outlook. As a novice nurse working grueling 12-hour night shifts, I found solace in our conversations.*
>
> *Mattie and I spent weeks together in the hospital, and we grew very close. I vividly remember the night she passed away. She gently placed her hand on my face and said, "You will be okay." Even as she neared the end of her life, she was offering me comfort. She died the following day, and I felt an immense sadness. At that time, I wondered how I would cope with repeated loss throughout my career.*
>
> *Thirty years later, I've learned to appreciate these thoughtful interactions with patients. I find solace in knowing that I've made a meaningful impact and done good work, despite the inevitable losses.*

What Do You Do for Self-care?

Fortunately, Erika has a very supportive husband. He understands her dedication to her patients and that her job is meaningful in her life. He supports her spending the kind of time that she does at work and all of the related aspects associated with that.

> *We find joy in simple pleasures like walking trails in the woods with our dog, spending time with friends, and savoring every moment.*

Happiness doesn't always come from grand gestures or global vacations. Sometimes it's about enjoying small things—whether that's working on a project in the yard, preparing a delicious meal together, or simply acknowledging the fragility of life. We cherish the time we have with each other because we never truly know what tomorrow may bring.

This really does capture mindfulness and self-care. It is appreciating the small things that refreshes our spirit and helps us to be present.

Meaning of Mindfulness in Oncology Care

When I think of mindfulness in oncology, to me it means being in the same space. Meeting patients and families where they are. It is important to convey important information such as prognosis, expectations for treatment, and honesty about impending life-threatening complications. Each conversation is different for each patient. Often patients will lead the conversation—"I am blessed. I'm not afraid. I've lived my life; I want to be comfortable. I want to be surrounded by my friends and family." Then too, others need to be led gently. As one human to another, it is hard to give news that will be hurtful, but patients and families deserve that kind of honesty so that they can make decisions and choices. I feel a sense of responsibility to help patients and family members to be prepared.

Erika honors her oncology experience and is very honest with her patients. It's a combination of respect and valuing their choices.

Wisdom to Share to Clinicians Going into Oncology

We hold an incredibly special place in our patients' and their families' lives. They look to us for comfort, whether through medicine or a simple hug. It's essential to be respectful of their feelings, especially since not everyone will always be on their best behavior due to pain, sadness, or misplaced anger. Sometimes, we absorb a lot emotionally, but it's important to remember it's not personal.

Patients often feel they need to be strong for those around them, and they may feel safest expressing their true emotions with us. There are times when we need to have thick skin, and other times when we simply need to acknowledge their feelings openly and reassure them that we are allies in their journey.

Most Impactful Part of Your Career?

Throughout my career, I've encountered countless experiences and situations that have profoundly impacted me. Each individual patient has contributed to shaping both my practice and my life.

One consistent pattern I've observed is that people often approach death in a manner similar to how they have lived. Those who have lived complex and chaotic lives tend to face their final moments with the same level of complexity and chaos.

CHAPTER 8

Misty Ceizyk, Medical Dosimetrist

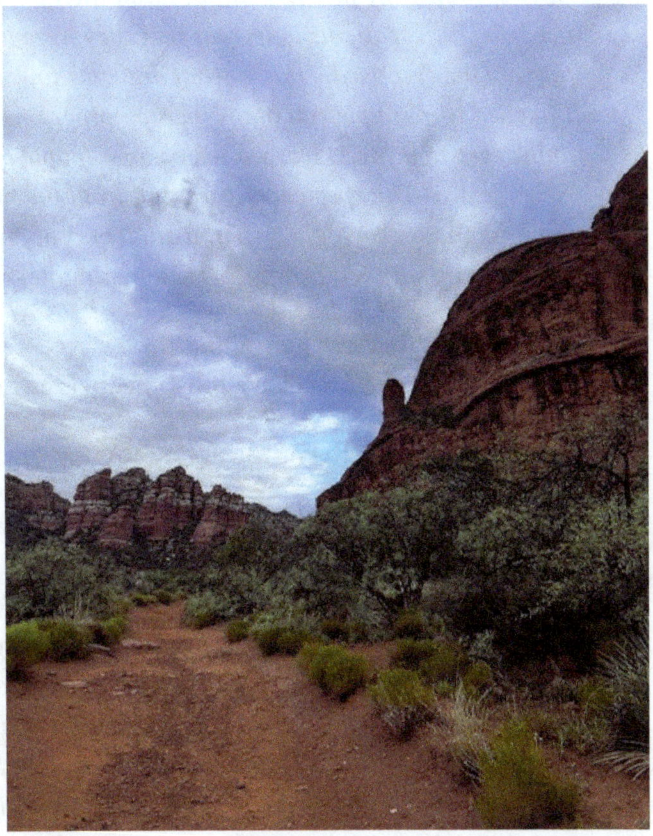

I feel very fortunate to have worked with Misty when I was interning at the Arizona Cancer Center. Immediately we connected as we were both young professionals. Misty was a radiation therapist who was very much in tune and supportive of her patients. I felt she really wanted to connect with her patients and give them the best support. She also was an integral part of the team and had a positive connection to the oncology team. One experience that I was really impressed with and always value was that Misty volunteered at a support group I created. It was for parents with cancer who were raising kids and their families, and Misty was instrumental in recruiting other radiation therapists to help me out. I felt validated in my work and trusted her to facilitate effectively.

Misty is a very empathic person, and it shows in her work with patients.

Why Did You Go into Oncology?

> *After high school, I played softball at a junior college in southern Illinois. There I was accepted and completed an educational program to become a general X-ray technologist. During this program, I decided to continue my radiological technology education in radiation therapy. I chose a career in radiation oncology because of the unique relationship I witnessed between radiation therapists and their patients. Unlike the other radiological technology specialties where you care for a patient one or maybe two times, as a radiation therapist you interact with your patients Monday to Friday and for weeks at a time. Before rotating through this specialty, I was worried the experience would be sad and depressing. After spending my first day in radiation therapy, I was pleasantly surprised. What I noticed about the patients I met was that they were upbeat, pleasant, and very appreciative of the care they received. This is what drew me toward radiation therapy. After X-ray school, I applied to multiple radiation therapy programs and ended up actually attending one I didn't even apply to. I was waitlisted on a couple of programs and accepted to University of New Mexico. Unexpectedly I got a call from the program director at a hospital-based program in Tucson saying they had a student drop out, leaving an opening in their program. "Is there any way you can fly to Tucson and interview for this position?*

And she just knew that was her calling, so she accepted the open spot, completed the program, sat for the board exam, and accepted a full-time therapy position. She is currently with the same team.

Misty worked directly with patients for almost 8 years before moving to medical dosimetry.

> *I am currently a medical dosimetrist, which is subsection of radiation oncology. I started my career as a radiation therapist in an academic medical center. Within a radiation oncology department, you have a group of professionals working together to care for patients. The radiation oncology team consists of radiation oncologists, nurses, medical physicists, medical dosimetrists, radiation therapists, and other healthcare professionals. Radiation therapists are the people who deliver the treatments on the linear accelerators. Medical dosimetrists generate the treatment plans behind the scenes. Medical physicists work closely with the medical dosimetrists, physicians, and therapists. They are responsible for machine quality assurance and patient safety.*

In our conversation, one prominent observation that I made was that Misty's career path first began working directly with patients. Her experience as a radiation therapist allows her to create treatment plans while considering all aspects of her patient's needs. She creates patient plans to the best of her ability with the chief aim of reducing side effects of treatment and contributing to the best possible outcomes. This intimate experience of connecting with her patients allows for her to do her best work as a medical dosimetrist.

What Is Your Personal Meaning from Oncology?

I think it's just that, what we do is truly impactful. Our daily efforts really do impact the patient and, if done well, with care and compassion, it can make a very positive difference in their experience.

What Insight Did You Gain from Your Work?

Self-advocacy and a good support system are crucial for patients who are navigating their journey through cancer care. I have learned to practice this in my own healthcare and my family's as well.

Memorable Moments to Share

Early in my career, our department would host a yearly holiday celebration. I always looked forward to this. Our patients were always so appreciative, and it was the one time we were able to give back to them in a different way. All the employees would make food for that day, and we would have local businesses contribute as well. With the help of our social working department, we would identify any patients in financial need during the holidays and support them through employee gift donations. That's memorable, for sure. We all looked forward to that.

I was running the Tucson half Marathon one year, when I happened to look over my shoulder to see a young man running alongside me. I thought he looked familiar and wondered if I knew him? And sure enough, he was a patient that we treated during the holidays when he was young boy. He was a week out of a bone marrow transplant and running in 13.1-mile run! We chatted for a moment and then he ran on toward the finish line. "Oh, my gosh, how incredible!" I felt emotional, I was very thankful at that moment to have shared in a small part of his journey, which was amazing. He would go on to inspire others and to be included in a Lance Armstrong book. He became an advocate for others with cancer and raised thousands of dollars for pediatric cancer research.

Another memorable moment was meeting a little girl we treated for a benign brain tumor when she was in kindergarten. From time to time, we would treat patients on a weekend day for one reason or another. One Saturday I came in to work to treat this little girl. I had been treating her since she started her treatments so had seen her parents every day she came in for treatment. There was a local jumping castle place for kids in town, and I thought how fun would it be for her to go. Somehow, we got to talking about it, and her parents thought it was a great idea, so I met her and her parents there. I spent time talking with her family enjoying watching her get to be regular kid for few hours. She is now 34 years old and though her life is full of struggles as result of her disease, she is one of the most positive people I know. She loves sharing her artwork that she found a love for her back when she was first diagnosed and loves watching Everyone Loves Raymond. My husband and I are blessed to have been able to watch her grow up over the years, attend her art shows, and even watch her strut her stuff in a charity fashion show. She and her mother have become part of our extended family. I will always be very thankful I was able to treat her on that Saturday.

What Do You Do for Self-care?

For self-care I enjoy running and group fitness classes.

How Do You Handle Sadness and Grief?

It's been so long since I worked directly with patients. I feel like you can kind of distance yourself from the patient and the emotions of what they are dealing with when you're just working with their CT scans and not seeing them in person. When something does come that is upsetting, like seeing a patient that comes back multiple times for treatment or hearing of a patient with a poor outcome, I definitely feel sad. I try to acknowledge my emotions at the time they arise. It is also sometimes helpful to talk to coworkers as they have similar experiences and offer great support. A few times I've written some things down just to kind of help me move through what I am feeling. Overall, I just try to focus on the positive contributions we are making and not as much about every outcome.

And then, when you were working directly with the patients, did you like attending funerals? How did you have closure in that way, or did you?

I never attended a patient's funeral, but years ago we did have a list of patients that had passed and though it was sad look through, in a strange way it gave me a bit of closure reading the names and knowing their pain and suffering was over. I would say, just running, exercising, and spending time with my family helps me cope with that.

Meaning of Mindfulness in Oncology Care

Being mindful of what patients may be experiencing and knowing that they have many things that they're dealing with. I may see only their physical disease on a CT scan, but there are many other aspects to consider. They may be receiving other treatments, have outside obligations, and social needs that may affect when they can come in for treatment. Patients may have other medical conditions that can limit how they can lay on our treatment table or the amount of time they can lay still. These are all things to keep in mind when developing a patient's radiation treatment plan.

What Have You Personally Brought to Oncology Care?

As a radiation therapist, I brought a smile, compassion, and a genuine interest in my patients' life. I recall many patients, in addition to talking about how they were feeling each day and how treatments were going for them, wanted to talk about their life outside of cancer. I found getting to know our patients was one of the most rewarding parts of my career. As a medical dosimetrist I bring my experience delivering radiation therapy treatment and treatment planning skills I have developed over the years. The quality of our treatment plans can directly relate to the side effect our patients experience during treatment.

Oh, wow! Yeah, so that's the difference between dosimetry and therapy.

I definitely miss the patients and value the years I spent as a therapist. Both careers are excellent and play an important role in the radiation oncology team. I do enjoy treatment planning, and I definitely like the fact that we can positively affect how our patients feel physically through our plans.

Wisdom to Share to Clinicians Going into Oncology

While a career of any type in oncology has its challenging days, the good days far outweigh the bad ones. Radiation oncology professionals are amazing caring individuals.

I believe it was really beneficial to treat on the machines before I became a dosimetrist. Even if you only treat on the machines for few years before moving into dosimetry, it will make a difference in the dosimetrist you can become.

How Do You Rationalize Cancer?

I am not sure how to rationalize cancer; it's unfortunately part of life we have little control over.

What Has Been the Most impactful Part of Your Career?

The most impactful part of my career as a dosimetrist takes place behind the scenes, every day creating the best possible plans keeping the dose to normal structures as low as reasonably achievable. Working in radiation oncology has been a very impactful career. It has rewarded me with wonderful relationships and hundreds of memories. Some of my coworkers are like family and past patients have felt like friends. My career has shaped my life.

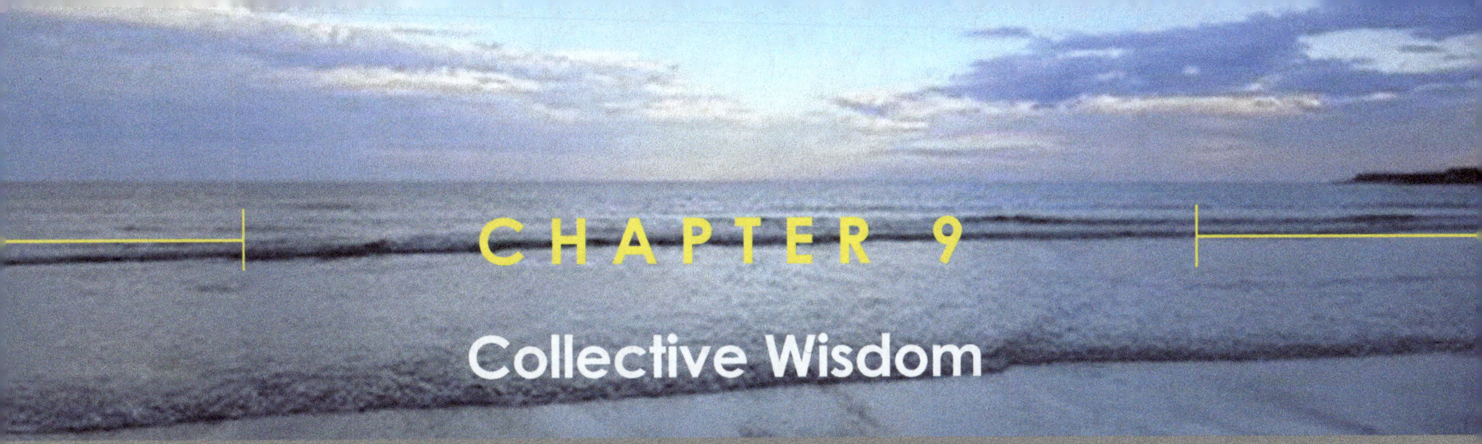

CHAPTER 9

Collective Wisdom

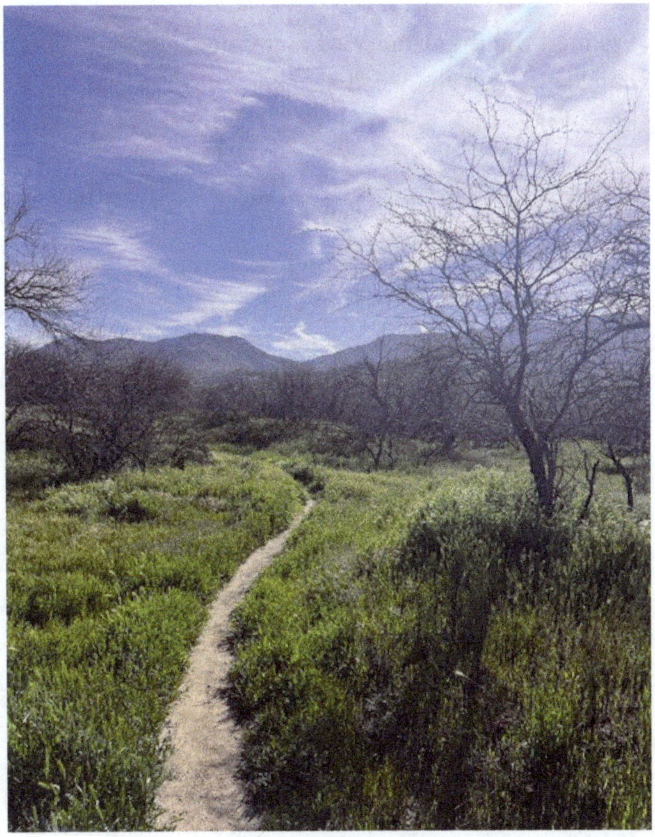

It was important to me to allow for other voices in oncology to be represented in this book. I recognize how different professionals want to share their input for this book and have the flexibility of just completing the questions in their own time and space. By offering this option, I was able to collect their wisdom together for inspiration.

I feel honored to have attended *American Psychosocial Oncology Society's conference a few years back. I was really fortunate to have met amazing colleagues across the United States providing exceptional psychosocial support to patients. I wanted to be able to include any members who were interested in participating.*

This chapter integrates different professionals from all over the country, and their wisdom is valuable.

Laura Hagerty, MSW, Oncology Social Worker

1. Why did you go into oncology?

I always had a desire to work in healthcare and was drawn to oncology as it's an area of healthcare where long-term relationships can be fostered with patients and families. It's a particularly rewarding area of practice as we work with patients with a broad range of needs at a very overwhelming time in their lives. Additionally, I find that oncology health providers are such compassionate and motivated humans on the earth. I enjoyed working alongside such fine people!

2. What insight did you gain from your work?

I gained the importance of enjoying each and every moment of life as I know how too well how quickly life can change. I also know how important it is appreciating the people in my life and to let them know that they are loved.

3. How do you handle the loss, sadness, and grief?

I would like to say it got easier for me, but it did not. I tried to embrace the feelings of sadness as a reflection of my connection and caring. I also tried to compartmentalize my feelings to minimize the impact on my personal life.

4. Memorable moments to share?

Oh, so many memorable moments, most of which involved end-of-life moments. The hardest moments are often when the family member has to leave their deceased loved one for the first time. One of the most impactful moments was taking a deceased baby boy from his mother's arms, wrapping him in a blanket, then carrying him to the morgue where I literally walked this baby into the refrigerator and handed him off to the mortician. Some of my sweetest memories and greatest honors were witnessing the love and dedication families offered their loved ones. How absolutely brave and caring they were despite their fear and sadness.

5. What do you do for self-care?

I exercise regularly, have a caring and supportive family, and have friends that "get" what I did for a living.

6. Meaning of mindfulness in oncology care?

In the cancer center where I work, mindfulness was incorporated into our care, and we offered many resources in this regard. In my role I taught my patients relaxation breathing techniques and stressed the importance of "be here now."

7. What have you personally brought to oncology care?

I aimed to bring compassion to my practice with an emphasis on advocating on behalf of my patients and families. I enjoy program development and utilized these skills to address patient and family needs within my work setting.

8. Wisdom to share to clinicians going into oncology?

Maintain boundaries, love but protect your heart, never work harder than your patients/families, encourage independence, accept people where they are (not where you think they should be), create a big and meaningful life outside of your work, ask for support when needed, and take care of yourself.

9. What does your specific profession bring to patients?

My profession brings a systems perspective to care. In the healthcare setting, it's vital to remember how a diagnosis impacts the patient, their family, and their community. In a blink of an eye, literally everything changes. Social workers are generally the one team member whose job it is to acknowledge that impact and assist in whatever way is possible. Advocacy is also a key role for the oncology social worker.

10. Most impactful part of your career?

I had the most rewarding career. It was a true calling for me, and, while I witnessed many difficult events, I also witnessed healing and growth. I loved working with the patients, families, and my colleagues. I can't imagine a better job for me.

Amy Clara

1. Why did you go into oncology?

Someone else saw the potential in me. I was working in Primary Care/Internal Medicine and was looking for a health psychology specialty. I had two mentors suggest looking into the world of oncology, but it seemed more niche than I was prepared for. In my search for my next career opportunity, I met with Dr. John Gilbert, a pillar in the psychosocial oncology community. In one phone call, I went from radical transparency "I don't think I could do it," to optimistically curious. If it wasn't for those two mentors and Dr. Greer, I wouldn't be at MGH nose-deep in the world of psychosocial oncology.

2. How do you handle the loss, sadness, and grief?

I connect with colleagues both in and out of the system. I have two amazing psychologist-friends from graduate school who practice far away from the world of health psychology but are more than familiar with the grief and despair that come with caring for suffering people. My in-house crew at the hospital are incredibly supportive. I text, I share, and I consult. I also cry a lot. I cry when I get the "gray box" after opening my patient's chart and it says "... Is deceased, do you wish to continue?" And later, I light a candle and say good-bye. I write their name on the matchstick and keep them in a jar in my closet. About 1 to 6 months later, I write a note to their loved ones, usually the spouse or adult children.

3. Memorable moments to share?

While sitting in a very serious session with a very serious young man who was being treated for GBM, my phone randomly started my Spotify and started to play Saweetie's "Tap In." It felt unprofessional and embarrassing; after he died, when I was connecting with his wife I mentioned this moment, and she laughed and told me he, in his diligent note-taking of our sessions, had written down the incident with an exclamation point. Human-to-human moments in the midst of very serious cancer moments are priceless.

4. What do you do for self-care?

I avoid cancer, suffering, and death-related content outside of work. I watch trashy TV, find interests outside of my work (baking, running, music), and engage in purpose that has nothing to do with my work-world (teaching older adults how to meditate and stay hydrated). I make sure that if I need to walk away, I can.

5. What have you personally brought to oncology care?

I like to call myself a "personality hire," but my director and mentors have told me to stop. I bring a face and space that is safe enough for people, patients, colleagues, trainees, to unload. I bring organization and collect resources so there's less precious time sending those "Does anyone know a [resource] for [cancer-related supportive care need]?" emails.

6. Wisdom to share to clinicians going into oncology?

Join us. But bring tissues and a water bottle.

7. Most impactful part of your career?

Watching my colleagues. They astound me to no end in their vulnerability and efforts to keep pursuing the best care.

The patients and their loved ones—everything expands in the space between diagnosis and the end, treatment, death, or otherwise. Anyone in this field will be humbled by witnessing the worst and best experiences of humankind.

8. Anything else to share?

A well-devised metaphor can be life-changing.

Share what you're thinking and feeling with your patients (selectively, yes, but be brave, join them in the mud puddle).

Oncology is not your average specialty; it will change you.

Ethan, Psychologist

1. Why did you go into oncology?

I went through cancer treatment as a child, and as I went through my doctoral training I became attached to the subject.

2. How do you handle the loss, sadness, and grief?

By having positive and enjoyable things to engage in outside of work.

3. Memorable moments to share?

While running a group, helping members through the grief related to the death of a group member.

4. What do you do for self-care?

Religion, hobbies, and a good social life.

5. What have you personally brought to oncology care?

Personal experience, strong clinical skills.

6. Wisdom to share to clinicians going into oncology?

Families are important, but the patient is the client.

7. Most impactful part of your career?

Helping clients adjust after surviving.

Gina M. Wendt-Blasing, Psycho-oncology Therapist, Cert. Exec. Coach, MS, LCMFT

1. Why did you go into oncology?

A variety of reasons: (A) Experienced my own cancer, stage 1 cervical, 1992. (Now, I say a piece of cake compared to all of those I've worked with. At the time, though, it was a tad scary.) (B) Volunteered at Duke University back in early 1990s on the adult cancer ward. Liked it. (C) Volunteered since 2008 as Psychotherapist/Speaker for a local Cancer organization. (D) In 2019, journeyed with my Dad, every step, through his cancer and death. (I'm an only child. He was my Dad, my brother, and friend/confidant.)

Also, I have always been in healthcare. BS Biology undergraduate. Hired with Eli Lilly Pharma in late 1980s (9 years). Then Roche Diagnostics middle/upper management (7 years). Then, ran two nonprofit medical clinics. I obtained my MS LMFT in 2008.

So, why did I go into oncology? Oncology got into me, ha! I want to listen to patients with cancer, journey with them, give them hope, help them recognize their resilience and navigate this "Terrain of Pain." Help them know that even in suffering, and often a terminal diagnosis, life can still hold meaning. Life can be lived, memories made. I also love helping the families of cancer patients. Overall, it is a privilege and honor journeying with them. Listening to their stories, their fears, their hopes. Helping them to create the legacy they want to leave to their loved ones. Helping them to know they matter and their life matters. They are heard, respected, and loved.

2. How do you handle the loss, sadness and grief?

My faith as a Christian gives me great strength, comfort, and hope. When a patient dies, I reflect on what I appreciated about them. I try to let them know all throughout our journey by sending them cards, notes, and verbally. In my personal life, my maternal aunt died from breast cancer, my paternal grandpa from bladder cancer. Recently, my dad in 2019, from small-cell lung cancer, my godmother in January 2024 lung cancer, and my first best friend and cousin, Quinn, died from colon cancer February 2024. (On March 2, 2024, both my mom and my mother-in-law died. Though, not of cancer, both had dementia and were 83 & 91, respectively.)

The truth is, as one of my current patients stated on his first appointment, "We are all terminal." Not to sound hard or harsh, by any means, but to understand that this life is temporary; we will all die of something at some point. So, let's learn to live life today. I keep my heart open to grieve and to be sad, when necessary/appropriate. I cry. I remember. I cry. I pray. I get good sleep, as much as possible. I give myself permission to enjoy life in honor of those who have died. I also use rituals to help me grieve. As previously shared, my mom and mother-in-law died on March 2nd. Yes, the same day, in separate nursing homes. Currently, we are preparing my mom's home to sell. I have taken my time to go through all of her things, while reminiscing (and crying). I have kept many things and bequeathed other items to my family. It is a labor of love and helps me grieve in a healthy way. I wrote a poem for her obituary, with her permission before she died. Writing is grief relief for me!

3. Memorable moments to share?

There are many, I will share four. (A) Approximately 7–8 years ago, a 58-year-old male patient was going through radiation treatments. High anxiety, fear of open spaces, fear of closed spaces. However, he was dedicated to working through his anxieties, fears, and panic. He did his homework, though, challenging at times. He successfully got through all of his radiation treatments and was declared cancer free. He sent me notes and texts for years after graduating therapy, every time he would get a favorable test/PSA. (B) At about that same time, I began seeing a 70+-year-old female with brain cancer. She said, "My daughter told me I would need to learn to be a human being versus a human doer." She explained that she was having to learn to just BE as she did not have the energy to DO a lot anymore. "I used to be up and down running around doing lots of things every day. Now, I am slowing down and do not know how to do this." I enjoyed hearing the goal she had, transition from "Human Doer" to "Human being." (C) Another patient, a fun, feisty 50+ female, during her second appointment, expressed tearful emotion at the thought of losing her hair during chemo. She said, "I feel out of control." After we discussed that we can learn to assume control of what we think, how we manage emotions, and how we choose to behave, this therapist said to her, "And, of course, you could take control in another way" (I paused, lifted eyebrows, cocked my head). She hesitated, processing my words and facial gestures, and responded, "Noooo .... are you saying? (then she cracked up laughing) .... Are you saying shave my head!?" I said, "YYYYES!" She read my mind. We both cracked up laughing and then seriously discussed the pros and cons. I assured her that I was just offering yet another way to feel like she will still have choices. "You have a voice and a choice on this journey." She shows up to her third appointment … yep, you guessed it, with a shaved head! She said, "It is so freeing to have done this!" I reminded her that SHE TOOK CONTROL over her cancer and decided to shave before the cancer could take her hair. At the end of our session, I walked her to the door, as I routinely do, and said, "You are fun, my Dear, I will see you in two weeks." She turned around, threw her arms around me and hugged me, for what seemed like 30 seconds. This was an unexpected surprise. She said, "Thank you, thank you. Thank you." That gesture stayed with me for several days, and each time I recalled it, I smiled. She did not show up for her next appointment. I texted her several times, offering to reschedule if she did not feel well, or was delayed at another appt. Never received a response. This bothered me. I called her, no answer. She had not listed an emergency contact. I knew she would get a hold of me. Found out that she had died from her cancer about a week after our last appointment. It was aggressive. (D) My fourth story is about a female, 60+. Creative, spicy, intelligent, witty, and optimistic. She came to me one-and-a-half years ago, sharing that she had a recurring cancer, stage 4. She was in a struggle emotionally, of course. She would say, "This is what I am going to die from." She shared her fears of dying, her regrets from the past. Today, she is going strong, resuming creative hobbies, very involved with family, realistic outlook, making many more memories. She has what seems like boundless energy. She says, "I'm living today!" I teased her at her last appointment, "I think you've been misdiagnosed; you don't have a terminal illness." She smiled, "Oh, but I do." And she does. And then she reiterates that she's alive today and living today! She is an exceptional woman with an optimistic view of today and all that it has to offer.

4. What do you do for self-care?

I write. I read. I send a lot of greeting cards to those I love and care for. I take vitamins/supplements. I take long Epsom salt baths, on occasion. I have frequent great discussions with my husband, who I met in third grade (51 years, best friends, only 28 years married). I spend time with family, mostly, and friends for dinner. Meet another psychotherapist/friend monthly for lunch. I pray daily. Devotions and Bible study. I implement my faith with trust. I deep-breathe all throughout the day, and longer in a quiet place, when needed. Drink 2 to 3 quarts of water/day and of course LOTS of coffee in a.m. I make sleep a priority, even though I have my struggles sleeping, on occasion. (CBT-I trained, so I know the tricks.) I am in the process of resuming exercise: stationary bike, occasional walking. Considering resuming swimming. (I am a former athlete from elementary through college.) Worked out routinely up to the age of 50. Old joints now hurt. And a not-so-successful hip replacement at 56, two knee surgeries in my 20s. I am now turning 61. I'm out of habit working out, so reclaiming this habit! My saying for this? "It's easy to suffer, change is tougher!" AND I LAUGH, A LOT! My husband was class clown and still is. We find humor in a lot of things, even during the most significant of times. I also watch comedians on Dry Bar when I need a good BeLLa! (Belly Laugh).

5. What have you personally brought to oncology care?

Experience. Knowledge. Compassion, Emotional Intelligence. Resilience. Dedication. Endurance. HUMOR. And a desire to learn from my patients.

6. Wisdom to share to clinicians going into oncology?

Ponder your reasons and objectives for this decision. There are all kinds of ways of helping. This type of "helping" can be draining and sad. Evaluate your health, overall, and your resilience. Put priority on SELF-CARE! What are your thoughts about death/dying ... can you talk about it fluently? Are you afraid of death? If so, get that worked out before endeavoring this specialty area. Consider that there will be a lot of suffering with patients, endurance is key on this journey. Also, the human spirit is precious and must be recognized. Having said all of this, oncology is a wonderful arena. I have met some of the most resilient, wonderful people/patients, and dedicated clinicians. I am inspired, daily, by all of them and did not expect this when I endeavored oncology. We NEED more dedicated, stellar clinicians in oncology. So, WELCOME! It can be a journey of blood, sweat, tears, fears, spears, sears ... and CHEERS! It is a worthy and worthwhile endeavor.

7. Most impactful part of your career?

Knowing my patients know that I care about them, that I will listen to their deepest fears and thoughts. Earning their trust. Helping them gain resilience on such a tumultuous journey. Helping them find meaning in the face of uncertainty. Observing them gain hope is priceless.

8. Anything else to share?

Bless you, Sarah, for writing this and for allowing me and others to give input. I wish you the absolute best!

Xiomara Rocha-Cadman, CL, Psychiatrist/Psycho-oncologist

1. Why did you go into oncology?

I decided to pursue psycho-oncology after I lost my sister to breast cancer at the age of 32.

2. How do you handle loss, sadness, and grief?

I have developed many tools throughout the years. I also run half marathons and full marathons, some to raise money for cancer research.

3. Memorable moments to share?

Being with my patients throughout their cancer journey and learning from their life lessons.

4. What do you do for self-care?

I travel, write, and run.

5. What have you personally brought to oncology care?

Psychotherapy and psychopharmacology through either one-to-one encounter, support group for patients, and group for caregivers and for medical staff.

6. Wisdom to share to clinicians going into oncology?

Being present and attending to our patients. Stay with them in the moment and listen to our patients.

7. Most impactful part of your career?

Mentoring the new generation and learning from my patients.

8. Anything else to share?

I feel honored every time a patient allows me to enter their private space. It is a gift they provide us when sharing their life lessons, fears, and reflections.

CHAPTER 10

Inspired Creation

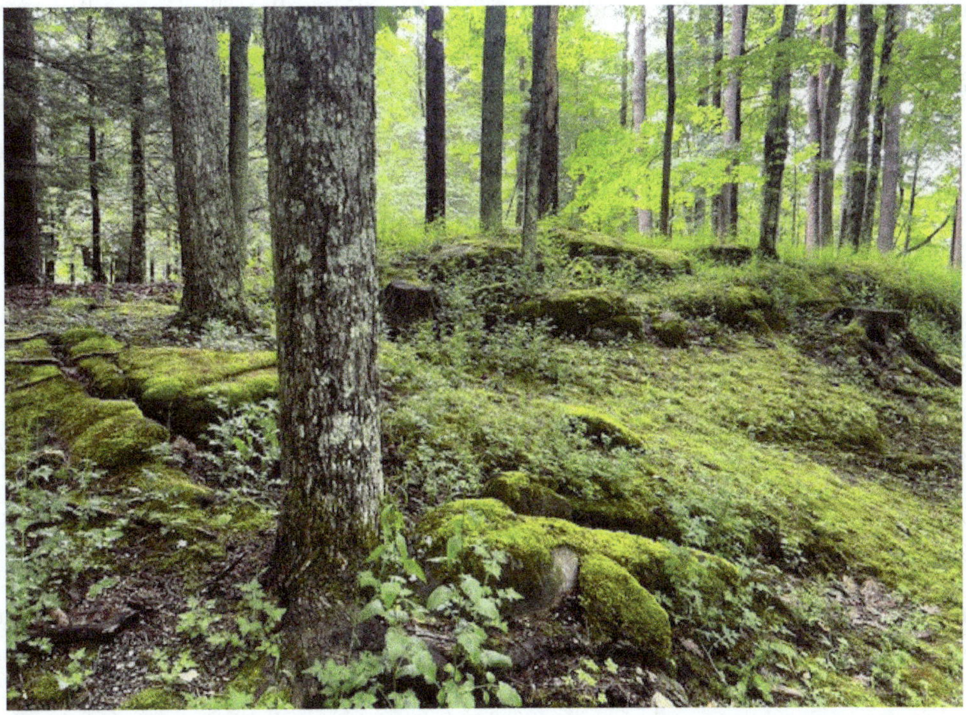

Vision

This book was really created to answer questions I had always wondered about oncology providers. I know from my experience that working in oncology provides such profound meaning in my life. And throughout my career meeting colleagues with the same dedication, I always wanted to ask them these questions. Understanding the impact of the purpose of our work has always been important to me. So, any chance to connect and comprehend their purpose, I took it. Therefore, this book really stemmed from the curiosity to know more about the impact.

To be able to conceptualize this book has been an evolving process. It stemmed from my mom's current oncologist who I had worked with at the start of my career. And now being in the caregiver position, I began to really wonder the influence of the work.

Then when I attended Integrative Health Summit at University of Arizona this past year and met John Kabat-Zinn, I began to really dream about this book. Not sure how or why, but I knew I needed to create this conversation for new professionals going into oncology. That these stories of influence needed to be a foundation available to new practitioners.

And being very mindful in my decisions but also letting the book and experience guide me has been a valuable process of learning for me. To be able to connect the oncology, mindfulness, and social work is a dream to me. To culminate these really powerful connections allowed me to really be present and learn from those who participated. To be able to make it mine while being encouraged makes me really proud of this project. There are so many lessons that I have learned from the process.

Being able to know that these stories are going to guide others in profound discussions makes me proud.

Interviews

The time spent with each clinician connecting to them in a very intimate experience of their careers was such a blessing. Not only did I learn from their stories, but I also felt a deep connection to my experiences in oncology. This validation of essential meaning was meditative. It brought up emotions and thoughts that expanded my capacity of understanding of the work we do.

Another component was the ability to validate and honor their experience. I feel I was able to be very present and welcoming and allowing them to reflect in a way that many had never experienced.

It was an emotional experience to be present and just listening to their stories. And the time to give them to honor their experience was to just be present with their words. I wasn't expecting how meaningful it would be for them to share it. My vision allowed for them to be honored by educating others.

Once I completed my first interview, I knew I had to allow for them to edit the chapters. I wanted them to be able to be proud of their expression of the story. It was important to me to give them that time and space to make sure it captured their experiences.

These interviews will always be a very humbling part of my career.

Collective Inspiration

Allowing oncology practitioners to be included in another storytelling option was an evident part of this book. It allowed for another outlet of expression for these individuals to make an impact to our psychosocial care.

Personal Impact

Various lessons that I didn't anticipate met me throughout this entire process. I truly feel they are gifts of being present and mindful of this experience. I was open to the process and took space and time to listen and learn.

One of the most inspiring lessons was the emotional connection I had from the interviews. I assumed that since I knew each clinician I would maybe just hear a summary of their experiences. I also assumed they would answer in a certain way based on what I knew from them. But that was not the case. I learned so much and I heard more stories of connection rather than of accomplishments.

It was a validating experience to hear each of them thank me for the experience. I really believed that they were doing me the favor of their time and sharing. But the interviewers really experienced personal value and meaning. My ability to listen and be present allowed for deep appreciation of their experiences.

It is evident throughout this book that oncology clinicians view their career as personal meaning and their work in life provides them with meaning and purpose.

I love that I created this dream and then was able to be present in each of the steps of accomplishment. I feel this book is the foundation of positive changes that I can create from my visions of how to positively inspire others.

Thank You

I want to sincerely thank Hannah and Vera from Kendall Hunt Publishing for their expertise and encouragement.

www.ingramcontent.com/pod-product-compliance
Lightning Source LLC
LaVergne TN
LVHW060454061126
851857LV00016B/1822